The Natural Cure to Your Migraine Headache –

What the Big Drug Companies Don't Want You to Know

4th Edition

By Andrew P. J

Table of Contents

Foreword to the 4th Edition

These are exciting times. This book is now in its third
year and fourth edition. New changes are coming
along at a rapid pace. Hence, the need for frequent
updates.

Migraine headache treatment for women is undergoing
a revolution of sorts. Since I first wrote the initial
edition back in January of 2006, we were using the
experience gained in treating our patients at the
Women's Health Institute of Texas located just outside
Houston, Texas.

What makes this 4th edition different from the last
edition is the addition of three new major
recommendations. Previously we recommended the
combination of bio-identical progesterone with
magnesium. This was successful by itself but we
learned we could do even better.

Based on shared information with other pioneers in the
field, new world-wide experience and the latest
research earlier in 2008, we are adding three new
recommendations consisting of Krill Oil, Iodine and
Vitamin D3 for a total of five items to rid your migraines.

We have also been successful in consolidating our
recommendations on supplements to just a couple of
manufacturers. In the past, my book purchasers were
scurrying around dealing with multiple vendors of
recommended products. Now it should be much more
convenient.

Over the last three full years, we have had the pleasure
of getting feedback from thousands of women, all over

the world, especially in the English speaking countries of the United Kingdom, Canada, Australia, New Zealand and of course, the USA.

Very soon, there will be a Spanish version of this book for Latin America and Spain. Migraine headaches do not respect language or political geographical boundaries.

The experience of women treating themselves from this guidebook has been especially rewarding with the mountain of testimonials these women send us via email on a daily basis. Only a small fraction of these testimonials are on our website, www.Migraine-Headaches-Information.com . The remainder are stacked up in a huge file on my desk.

We read every letter, every email and every testimonial that you send. We strive to answer each and every one of them. Sometimes we get behind. If we fall too far behind, just send it again to remind us and we will respond.

Our philosophy is to help women around the world end their nightmare with migraine headaches through natural measures and without having to deal with a frustrating and ignorant mainstream medical system. This book will teach you everything you need to know without having to see a doctor or require a prescription.

I am sure, like thousands of women before you, that you will be very pleased with your results.

Andrew Jones, M.D.

September, 2008

Introduction

Congratulations – on the purchase of my book that will help you to end your migraine headaches forever. You have taken the first step towards living a pain-free life.

Migraine headaches are controversial. Many people and doctors have definite opinions on them, but exceedingly few offer up anything for curing them. They can't cure them because they don't know how to. But I do – and I have been curing them for a long time. Read on and learn exactly how you can cure your migraine headaches once and for all.

If you are like my typical patient, you have been to 20 or 30 doctors over the years and taken numerous prescription medications. You have been prescribed anti-depressant medications, pain medications, anti-inflammatory medications, and more recently, triptan medications – like Imitrex®, Zomig®, Amerge®, Maxalt®, etc.

Of all of these medications, only the triptans have worked, but eventually, they seem to lose effectiveness and you end up switching brands and suffering numerous side effects almost as severe as migraines themselves along the way. Did I mention that you have to have a migraine attack already started (or on the way) to begin with before you start taking the triptans?

I have another group of patients who rarely see doctors and the few doctors they saw were their family physicians who either downplayed their migraines or were ineffective in their treatments. More often than not, they were mis-diagnosed as having tension headaches or sinus headaches. Either way, these patients just tend to give up on the mainstream medicine system altogether and learn to live with their migraines. This group tends to have fewer migraines than the first group and eventually just drop out of the medical system.

Both groups of patients still have severe, disabling headaches and regardless of the number or type of doctors that they have seen, have not been cured. These patients vary in the intensity, severity and frequency of their headaches. But, regardless of their experiences with the mainstream medical system, they are all desperate for a cure.

Well, I have a cure. And it is very simple and straightforward. It relies on normal human physiology that medical students were taught in their first year of medical school. It is safe. It is a combination of natural products which I will describe later in this e-book. It is also relatively inexpensive versus mainstream prescriptions and has no unpredictable nor unpleasant side effects. And nobody, I mean nobody, is out there in the mainstream medical community pursuing this avenue of treatment and cure.

What makes my approach to the cure of migraine headaches even better is the fact that most people have many symptoms above and beyond migraines that affect them. For example, many women have painful menstrual cycles, or PMS, or even infertility issues that most doctors do not even ask about when a woman comes in to see them complaining about her severe headaches.

All of these total body symptoms are related to one another in a big picture scenario that virtually all specialists in today's American medicine setting will miss. The narrow specializing doctors that people suffering with migraines are usually referred to have no idea about the relationship between these seemingly unrelated symptoms that are, in fact, all part of the same SINGLE problem.

The good news is that in my 20 years of private practice, I have managed to spend a lot of time with my patients and have asked a lot of questions about various health problems that were seemingly unrelated to the issues they have originally come to see me for. Having accumulated those years worth of observations, I have been able to put all of them together and discover that all of these symptoms are actually just consequential results from the same single problem.

For example, when we talk about migraine headaches, the classic description you have probably heard has to do with blood vessels in the brain that open up or dilate causing nerve irritation or inflammation to the nerves in the brain and spinal cord. This supposedly is the mechanism for the "aura" that frequently precedes the migraine and the skin sensitivity around well defined parts of the face and body.

I will go on and discuss this in much more detail later in this book, but let's say this mechanism is completely accurate. What then? What causes the blood vessels in the brain to dilate and cause inflammation or irritation to nerves in the first place? The answers are to follow.

An interesting story from the history books of medicine is the disease called scurvy. Three hundred years ago, crewmembers on ocean going ships sailed for months at a time on the open sea living off dry foodstuffs and fish. They had no fruit or vegetables. Many sailors were afflicted by scurvy, which is basically a severe deficiency of vitamin C.

Eventually, the British Navy figured out that if the crew were to eat limes during their long journeys that they would not get scurvy. It took three centuries to figure out the science, but they empirically noted it and treated the problem. Nowadays, every school kid in the world knows that vitamin C is found abundantly in fruit and even a small amount prevents scurvy.

The same type of approach follows for migraine headaches. People do not get migraine headaches because they are deficient in Effexor® or Imitrex® drugs. They get it because their bodies are deficient in certain substances called hormones and likely are deficient in certain nutrients. Later on I will tell you which ones in particular.

Read on for the most unique approach you have ever seen towards migraine headaches. Actually, this approach I employ was standard medical treatment more than 60 years ago. This was before the days when lab tests took over all diagnostics and moved the physician from asking questions, to just ordering tests and letting the tests tell him what was wrong.

The problem with the modern medicine approach is that most of the time, lab tests are not helpful enough. The ranges for "normal" are so wide and the fact that the body can compensate so well on the last 10 percent of a functioning organ mean that lab tests are virtually always normal except in people who are ready for the hospital or the early grave.

By then, the lab tests are usually too late. Modern medicine needs to return to its roots just like the British Navy doctors did – by observation. Although we may not have the exact scientific mechanism to explain to the smallest detail what causes migraine headaches, we can certainly employ the powers of observation and use what works to eliminate them altogether – for good.

Now, YOU will be the beneficiary of this approach. Just like the British Navy made its observations over the years and found out just how to prevent scurvy in its sailors, my progressive medical colleagues and I have discovered the **NATURAL SOLUTION** for curing migraine headaches preventing them from happening in the first place.

We have demonstrated a cure rate of 80% in patients with migraines, being especially effective in treating women. Why 80% and not 100%? Because there may be some overlap of more than one type of headache, with not all of them being migraines. Read on further to see how to determine what kind of headache YOU are suffering from.

How Common Are Migraines?

Depending on whose statistics you use, migraine headaches are found in about 10% of the population. Since women officially have three times more incidence of headaches than men, the number of females experiencing migraines approaches18%. As women approach the age of 35, the peak incidence of migraines increases to nearly 35% - nearly one in three!

These figures are consistent worldwide – and not just limited to the United States.

Earlier studies raised the issue that Asians experience far few migraines than Westerners. However, recent surveys seem to refute this finding. This is interesting – because it would seem to indicate that migraines are a universal human condition and not cultural or developmental phenomena.

It's also estimated another 5% of the worldwide population have migraine headaches but don't know it! These people have either incorrectly self-diagnosed their condition - or had their pain misdiagnosed by doctors as tension or sinus headaches.

Of all the people who experience migraine headaches, properly diagnosed or not, about 20% are supposed to have the "classical" aura type of migraine.

Migraines Much More Common Than Realized

In real practice however, my observations have shown migraine headaches are much more common in the general population than formerly reported. Twice as many women as previously thought, about 1 in 5, will experience at least one migraine in their life. But of those women, very few of them experience an aura.

Furthermore, official statistics indicate that 60-70% of women experience "hormonal" headaches - headaches based on their monthly cycle.

Again, my actual experience is that far more women experience migraine headaches tied to menstrual cycle changes than officially recognized. In all likelihood, this is due to external stimuli affecting the body – such as birth control pills and certain prescription medications.

Migraine Headaches Swelling Worldwide

What's even worse, migraine headaches seem to be increasing worldwide, especially over the last 50 years, and particularly in women. Preliminary observations indicate that virtually every family in America has at least one female member experiencing migraine headaches.

The Centers for Disease Control reported a 60-percent increase in the incidence of migraine headaches from 1980 to 1989. A Mayo Clinic study released in 1999 showed similar findings where migraine headaches in women increased 56 percent during the 1980s while the incidence of migraine headaches in men increased 34 percent during the same period.

The clinic's author speculated the reasons were four-fold:

- "Stress"
- A rise in the number of single-parent households

- An increase in the number of women in the workforce
- An increase in women who are dieting for weight loss

With all due respect to the Mayo Clinic, the Women's Health Institute of Texas believes in alternate explanations for the increasing incidence of migraines:

- Increased use of birth control pills since 1960
- Progressive exposure to "xenoestrogens" over the last 50 years
- Worsening dietary habits over the last 25 years

All three reasons certainly account for the disturbing uptrend in women's migraines. The last two reasons apply to men just as well as to women. The entire population is being exposed to high levels of xenoestrogens, and the dietary habits of both men and women have progressively declined - as evidenced by the ever-rising numbers in obesity.

Part of the dietary changes includes the nutritional devaluation of the food supply. You will read later on about deficiencies in iodine, magnesium and Vitamin D.

A proliferation of antibiotics and hormones added to animal feed ends up on your dinner plate. Also decades of soil depletion of crop farm land has led to a bankruptcy of nutrients and minerals in grains, fruits and vegetables.

What are Xenoestrogens?

Xenoestrogens are chemicals exhibiting estrogen-like activity. Estrogen is one of the main female hormones.

"Xeno" means foreign, so xenoestrogen simply means "a foreign estrogen." There are tens of thousands of chemicals that exert hormonal effects, with xenoestrogens exerting estrogenic effects.

Examples of xenoestrogens include pesticide residues on fruits and vegetables, hormone additives to grain fed beef and "gas off" from plastic water bottles.

Too much exposure to estrogen can cause numerous medical difficulties, manifesting as a myriad of "female" problems in women. These range from PMS, to uterine fibroids, to breast cancer. In men, these can range from gynecomastia (development of breast tissue) to prostate cancer.

Incidentally, this problem doesn't just involve humans. A recent article in "The Week" magazine cites estrogen-like contaminants being responsible for male fish in Maryland's Potomac River actually carrying eggs! What used to be a one in a million abnormality now affects 80% of the smallmouth bass population.

Migraine headaches used to be a known, but uncommon condition a century ago. Today, migraines have become a worldwide epidemic representing a public health issue that authorities are missing out on.

Migraine headaches in women usually go hand in hand with other "female" problems like PMS, uterine fibroids, ovarian cysts, irregular and painful periods, post-partum depression and various cancers. Surgical procedures, like hysterectomies, are so commonplace that about a half million women are getting them done on an annual basis in the US alone. Worldwide, hysterectomies are probably numbering in the millions.

It is not natural that all of these problems are occurring. Migraines, PMS and hysterectomies are not normal and should not be considered so. Something is driving this trend – and it is getting worse, not better.

Birth control pills are a huge contributor to this epidemic, but public health exposure to xenoestrogens is sufficient enough by itself, to cause problems. The combination of effects from birth control pills and exposure to xenoestrogens is a catastrophe spiraling out of control.

But at least you are taking one small part of this into your hands. You can control some parts of this. The treatment program that you are about to learn will enable you to overcome and escape the pandemic that is occurring worldwide in women.

Read on and be free of the migraine headaches that have plagued you so much in the past. Victory over migraines is imminent and in your grasp.

So Many Different Headaches – So Many Different Names

So many times I have heard patients saying things like:

"My doctor tells me I have a TENSION headache (or SINUS headache) (or CLUSTER headache) but why is it SO DISABLING?"

"What kind of headache do I REALLY have?"

And the answer is usually very simple:

Your TENSION (or SINUS) (or CLUSTER) headache might actually be a MIGRAINE headache!

<u>Primary Headaches</u>:

The fact is that there are numerous kinds of headaches: **tension**, **sinus**, **TMJ**, and **migraine** are the most common ones. These types of headaches are called <u>primary headaches</u> and we will discuss all of them.

I would say that although **tension headaches** fall into a general musculo-skeletal category, they may be caused by any one of four different mechanical pain generators. A mechanical pain generator is a trigger to tension headaches. The four different mechanical pain generators originate from:

- damaged muscles
- torn ligaments
- broken or bruised bones
- pinched or inflamed nerves

Usually, the source of tension headaches is readily identifiable – generally from some type of trauma or injury, like head trauma (concussion), whiplash, even sneezing or coughing too hard, or sleeping in an uncomfortable position. People can generally point to a particular day or event and recite exactly when their headaches started.

Sinus headaches are probably terribly overrated and over-diagnosed. The sinuses are located in the skull and facial bones and are very well localized. It should be easy to identify these headaches as a sinus origin when the cause is attributed to a cold or flu. Only in the event of fungal overgrowth of a sinus cavity after numerous rounds of antibiotics do sinus headaches become a problem.

Most doctors never consider the possibility that fungus or yeast can be present inside the sinuses and these can become a chronic problem. Children are the most likely to have these types of headaches after suffering from numerous rounds of ear infections, tube placement and multiple rounds of antibiotics or steroid use (like prednisone or medrol dose packs).

If you are having a hard time visualizing fungus or yeast in a sinus after the application of antibiotics for the "flu", just remember what frequently happens to a woman after she takes certain kinds of antibiotics. Quite often she will develop a vaginal yeast infection.

The same thing can happen in the sinuses. This is why we really don't want to prescribe antibiotics every time somebody has a cold. Antibiotics select out an overgrowth of yeast and the sinus is a difficult place to get rid of it.

Even so, headaches from muscle contraction, head injury or sinus infection are not nearly as painful or debilitating as a migraine. They never have any neurological symptoms like tingling, visual symptoms like flashing lights, numbness, and weakness in one side of the face or body, flushing, or an aversion to light (photophobia).

Temporomandibular joint **(TMJ) headaches** arise from a problem with the jaw. The jaw bone (mandible) is attached to the skull via two hinge joints just in front of each ear. These jaw hinge joints are called the TMJ joints. Damage, inflammation or irritation to either of these joints can cause significant headaches on the side of the head, inside and around the adjacent ear. Chewing or opening the mouth makes these headaches much worse.

Now, you may ask - what about migraines? Migraine headaches are the emphasis and main focus of this book and will be thoroughly discussed in subsequent chapters.

Secondary Headaches:

Other types of headaches are called secondary headaches. This means that some other disease in process is causing them. The worst one of these diseases is a brain tumor. Second on that list are vascular catastrophes like a burst berry aneurysm or a stroke.

Another sudden presentation of a secondary headache can be caused by meningitis or encephalitis which are both infections of the brain tissue. Bacterial meningitis can be lethal, whereas viral meningitis is usually recoverable. The presence of a triad of fever, stiff neck and severe headache needs to be evaluated in the emergency room quickly.

Brain tumors can be a cancer that begins in the brain or can be a metastatic cancer that went to the brain from some other source, like breast cancer. The headache from a brain tumor is occasionally the first sign of the cancer with a poor prognosis. Many times a seizure is soon to follow. Migraines are never associated with seizures.

In any event, secondary headaches are very bad news. If someone shows up in the emergency room with the "worst headache of my life", this needs to be taken very seriously and thoroughly examined. Migraines have to start at some point as the "worst headache of my life" and the initial onset needs to be evaluated to make sure that none of the devastating secondary headaches are present.

Ultimately, the secondary headaches are self-limiting. Unfortunately, they end relatively quickly either with death or recovery. They don't repeat themselves and are easily diagnosed.

Now, what about **migraines**? Here are the facts - approximately 1 out of every 10 people experience migraines. Yet, many people suffer needlessly because they don't recognize the symptoms that can accompany migraines. They also underestimate the impact that their headaches are having on their lives.

If you don't get the relief you need from your frequent bad headaches, you may have migraines. It is estimated that 14 million Americans and possibly 100 million people worldwide who suffer from migraines have not been diagnosed with migraines yet. Could you be one of them?

About 40% of all people with migraines are misdiagnosed as having other types of headaches. Even cluster headache, which is an incredibly severe headache, is actually just another form of a migraine headache.

Do YOU Have A Migraine?

Here is how you can determine whether what you're experiencing is actually a migraine:

If you experience any 3 or more of the following symptoms, you are highly likely to have migraines:

- Your headache feels like someone has stabbed an ice pick inside your brain
- Pain is usually one sided (but can be both sided, especially if present around the eyes)
- Your headache does not respond to regular over-the-counter painkillers
- Pain is pulsating, pounding, or throbbing
- Light and sound bother you a lot
- Pain worsens when you move or bend over
- Pain becomes so intense that you throw up or become nauseated
- You get dizzy just by turning your head (lying in bed)
- You feel that you have to lie down, go to bed, or withdraw to a quiet dark room
- Vision may be blurred, like a curtain comes down over your visual field in one or both eyes
- The headache can last from several hours to several days (or even weeks)

People with tension headaches or sinus headaches do not and never will have a <u>disabling</u> headache. Cluster headaches are just another type or subset of a migraine headache.

The key word here is **"DISABLING"**. If your "tension" or "sinus" headache is disabling, then you do not have a tension or sinus headache. You have a migraine. Only migraine headaches are disabling. The table above is a nice listing of symptoms, but the bottom line is if you have to stay home and lock yourself in a dark, quiet bedroom, then you have migraines.

If you are reading this e-book because of severe, debilitating headaches that are poisoning your life, do not respond to painkillers, and keep coming back over and over again; you are very likely to have migraines. People with standard tension or sinus headaches do not bother to look them up on the Internet. You are here because YOUR bad headaches are interfering with your life and you are looking for a way to fix that. If you keep suffering through tremendous pain along with other symptoms mentioned above, then you have migraine headaches. And yes, they CAN be cured once and for all.

What are Migraine Headaches?

Now that you have established that you really do have migraine headaches, just what is a migraine anyway? Ask 10 doctors and you will get 10 opinions. It just seems that nobody really knows.

Here are the symptoms commonly associated with migraine headaches:

- Your headache feels like someone has stabbed an ice pick inside your brain
- Pain is usually one sided (but can be both sided, especially if around the eyes)
- Your headache does not respond to regular over-the-counter painkillers
- Pain is pulsating, pounding, or throbbing
- Light and sound bother you a lot
- Pain worsens when you move or bend over
- Pain becomes so intense that you throw up or become nauseated
- You get dizzy just by turning your head (lying in bed)
- You feel that you have to lie down, go to bed, or withdraw to a quiet dark room
- Vision may be blurred, like a curtain comes down over your visual field in one or both eyes
- The headache can last from several hours to several days (or weeks)
- Part of your face goes numb
- Part of your face gets weak, just like with a stroke
- An arm or a leg gets weak, just like with a stroke

Some people can get a migraine without a headache! Some people can lose vision in one eye temporarily.

Doctors tend to divide migraines into two major categories: those with an aura and those without an aura. The ones with the aura are called "classical" migraines and the ones without an aura are called "common" migraines.

An aura is a pre-migraine sensation that can evoke visual symptoms of flashing lights, partial loss of vision, or some déjà vu type of sensation. These typically precede the onset of the headache by a few minutes to an hour. For those of you with these types of headaches this is your window of opportunity to take one of the Triptan medications in the hopes that you can ward off the dreaded migraine headache that follows.

But most people do not have the classical aura and have to deal with the onset of headache as it occurs. Then you start to worry about if this is going to be the "big one" or just a flash in the pan and you can avoid taking the expensive medications (from US$20 to US$70 per pill).

Other kinds of migraines listed by doctors include:

- Hemiplegic migraine – which consist of a stroke-like paralysis on one side of the body

- Opthalmoplegic migraine – which is mainly centered around the eye with pain and visual symptoms

- Basilar migraine – frequently confused with tension headaches with base of the head pain, neck pain and dizziness

- Benign exertional headache – headaches brought on by heavy physical activity like running

- Status migrainosus – this is the migraine headache that just doesn't quit. It can last for a week or even longer

It is also necessary to mention that although people can get very dizzy and nauseated from migraines, some other traumatic headaches can also elicit dizziness when a condition called **vertigo** is present.

Vertigo is an inflammation of the balance organs of the inner ears and is frequently involved after head trauma. However, vertigo will virtually always disappear after a certain amount of time – usually no longer than a few weeks at the most. Whereas, the migraine headache can perpetuate dizziness and nausea each time there is a headache.

Modern Migraine Headache Theories

There are a number of theories out there on what causes migraine headaches. The most popular is the one formulated by a neurosurgeon about 70 years ago when he was operating on a patient (who was awake during the procedure). Just a note on this part: there are no sensory nerves on the brain itself. So once the skull is opened, a patient can be awakened and the brain can be probed without any pain whatsoever.

Dr. Harold Wolff, a prestigious and influential headache researcher, held that the brain does not feel pain and that migraine symptoms resulted from a stress-induced constriction of blood vessels inside the brain and a dilation of blood vessels outside the brain.

In later years another theory became popular. This theory had to do with neurotransmitter modulation through an imbalance of serotonin and norepinephrine. A neurotransmitter is a chemical released by nerve cells that float from one nerve cell to another. Cell receptors pick up these neurotransmitters and cause the cell to change their electrical signals.

Both serotonin and norepinephrine also can circulate out in the bloodstream and affect organs and cells some distance away from the brain, too. When viewed in this manner, they are called hormones.

When they are acting like hormones a long way from the point at which they were produced and released into the bloodstream, they can affect any cell in the body. Other examples of hormones are thyroid, estrogen, progesterone, cortisol, insulin and testosterone. There is a system of balances in the body whereby the level of one hormone affects the level of other hormones.

The brain is a major modulator of hormones within the body largely through the hypothalamus and pituitary gland. These brain areas sense the amount of hormones in the bloodstream and can issue signals to the cellular manufacturers of these hormones to make more or less of them. When this traffic cop type of management breaks down, then imbalances result in body-wide symptoms.

Cortical Spreading Depression (CSD)

Another modern migraine theory embraces special imaging and magnetic brainwave studies that strongly suggest that Cortical Spreading Depression (CSD) forms the biological basis for the "negative symptoms" of a migraine aura.

From studying a particular type of migraine - **Familial Hemiplegic Migraine (FHM)** - recent findings have shown two genes are responsible for causing this symptom. These genes - which control the ion flow of calcium, sodium and potassium to the nerve cells - are damaged in people inclined to this type of migraine. It's believed this genetic mutation makes a person's neurons susceptible to CSD.

In essence, the nerve cells (or neurons) don't get properly "recharged" – resulting in diminished or depressed neural activity. Whatever the reason, this reduced activity slows down normal body functioning. If the affected neuron complex happens to control the sight centers (visual cortex) then visual disturbances or losses may occur.

However, as these neurons begin to react to or recover from the CSD, they may become hyper excitable, resulting in visual phenomena such as flashing lights and zig zag lines. (It's sort of like the neuron's compensate by rebounding and going into overdrive!)

This hyper excitability then activates the major nerve complex behind the eye (trigeminal nerve). This initiates migraine headaches by activating the highly pain-sensitive "dura mater" - the membrane sheet wrapping around the brain.

Currently, the mainstream medical community believes that serotonin and norepinephrine are the primary hormones involved in migraines. There is probably some truth to that theory and the medications they prescribe do indeed modulate the levels of those neurotransmitters.

But, my observations indicate that other hormones are involved as well. This is particularly evident in women. Women make up the vast majority of migraine sufferers. Conservative statistics state that women are three times more likely to have a migraine than men. My observations over the years show that women make up a much higher proportion than that.

Furthermore, of the women that have migraines, almost all of them (60 to 80 per cent, according to medical literature) experience migraines at a certain time within their menstrual cycles (hormone headaches). Usually these migraines occur in the week prior or in the two week timeframe consisting of the week of menses and the week preceding it.

Virtually every woman with migraines has some other type of a menstrual problem, like heavy and/or painful periods, irregular periods, PMS, uterine fibroids, swelling, etc. Most have thyroid deficiency problems as well. The younger women may not manifest thyroid problems until after the birth of their first child. Infertility is another big problem on this list.

Many women with hormone headaches also tend to get worse after starting to take birth control pills. Most women get temporary relief when they are pregnant.

All of this indicates that hormones, particularly the sex hormones in women, are strongly related to migraine headaches.

What Is the REAL Cause of Migraines?

OK, so I have teased you with the esoteric discussion of migraine causes and shown you all of the current theories. I have sprinkled in some of my observations. Now, you may rightfully ask, "Dr. Jones, can you just tell me what really causes my migraine headaches?"

In the preceding chapter we have touched on the topic of hormones. We talked about the two favorite hormones of the medical establishment – serotonin and noreprinephrine. Mainstream medicine's favorite medications are those imposed upon them by the big drug companies – anti-depressants and triptans (Imitrex®, Amerge®, Maxalt®, Zomig®, Avert®, Frova®, Relpax®). They are selling huge dollar amounts of drugs to treat serotonin and norepinephrine levels.

But – here is the **TRUTH**. The cause of migraines is NOT serotonin or norepinephrine. It is not cortisone. There may be a relationship with thyroid, however. There may be a significant relationship with estrogen. All of these are interrelated and play a role as they interact with one another, but they are NOT by themselves the root cause of migraine headaches!

The primary cause is a hormone called **PROGESTERONE**.

Actually, it is a deficiency of progesterone (or an imbalance in the ratio of progesterone and estrogen) that appears to be the root cause of migraine headaches – at least in women.

Stated another way, **it is an imbalance in the female sex hormones, progesterone and estrogen, that causes migraine headaches**.

Earlier in 2006, the world's leading academic authority on migraine headaches and their relationship to hormones, Dr. Vincent Martin, of the University of Cincinnati College of Medicine, Ohio, published in the Journal, Headache, a blockbuster review article in which he discusses a theory called "estrogen withdrawal".

This is a variation of the progesterone deficiency theory. He noticed in a couple of studies done by earlier researchers that large quantities of estrogen administered late in the menstrual cycle that were suddenly withdrawn seemed to precipitate migraine headaches.

This is precisely in the point of the menstrual cycle where progesterone is supposed to be produced in increasing amounts. When the progesterone fails to be produced in sufficient quantities, then the amount of estrogen that is still floating around is sensed by the body as excessive.

The levels of estrogen also fall off rapidly before the onset of menses. When this happens in an environment of insufficient progesterone, then this triggers a migraine.

Testing for Blood Levels of Hormones

When patients come into our clinic for an initial consultation and examination we have always tested for blood levels of multiple hormones: progesterone, testosterone, estrogen, cortisol and thyroid.

My medical colleagues and patients alike love to discuss various blood levels of hormones as if one were at an academy of science meeting with esoteric comments about a relatively higher or lower than normal result shown. But my observation has been that 95% of the time ALL blood testing is so-called "normal" – at least according to the laboratory's idea of what a normal range should be.

Hence the problem with blood level testing of hormones. They are nice to look at. They make a great source of conversation at follow-up doctor visits. But they really don't make a difference in the treatment plan.

In other words, they don't really affect the decisions or dosages in treating migraine headaches. Regardless of how "normal" the blood testing is, we are still going to treat you the same way.

Why is this? Several reasons:

The lab's "normal" range is too wide. Virtually all labs consider one standard deviation "outside" the normal range. Mathematically, this puts 95% of the population in the "normal" range and only 5% of people as "abnormal".

If one considers the paradigm that 50% of women over the age of 35, for example, are deficient in progesterone, that stands to reason that the lab is missing an additional 45% or so of "abnormals".

What is more important - a lab's opinion of what your normal should be compared to a large population sample or what your own body considers to be a deficiency today relative to what your body experienced 10, 15 or 25 years ago?

In other words, the lab may say that you are "normal", whereas your body now has only half of the circulating progesterone (or estrogen, or thyroid) that you had when you were 20 years old.

What we don't have are the blood levels of what you had when you were 20 years old to compare back to. It is the relative difference inside your own body that makes all the difference.

So this is why blood testing is not important and not necessary in making recommendations for hormone replacement, at least in terms of managing migraine headaches. And this is why as you read further on in my treatment recommendations that you will see nothing about getting blood tests or hormone levels checked.

Now, let's take a closer look at **PROGESTERONE DEFICIENCY** in women – the **REAL CAUSE** of their migraines.

Sex Hormones – The Silent Culprit

Progesterone is one of the main sex hormones in women. Actually, both men and women have progesterone circulating around in their bodies, but women just have a lot more of it.

Progesterone is a sex hormone produced largely by the ovaries. It is a counter-balance to estrogen, also largely produced by the ovaries. The adrenal glands can also manufacture sex hormones, but the ovaries are the primary production facility.

Progesterone and the other sex hormones are carried in the bloodstream all over the body. Every cell in the body, whether it is part of the uterus, heart, liver, eyeball or brain has a special progesterone receptor. This means that as progesterone (and all other hormones) are circulating throughout the body, every cell on every organ can be affected.

The sex hormones therefore are not just concerned with the sexual organs (uterus, breasts, ovaries, vagina), but all other organs are affected as well, especially the brain.

If there is a deficiency in progesterone, then every cell in every organ system can sense that. This is why a woman with a progesterone deficiency can have many, many different health issues. For example, a woman with a progesterone deficiency can have numerous problems with her menstrual cycle ranging from heavy periods to infertility. Virtually every woman with migraine headaches has some menstrual problems as well.

The name Progesterone is derived from the base word – "gestation", or "pro gestation". This means that progesterone is responsible for the promotion and maintenance of pregnancy.

It is secreted by the ovary in the second half of the menstrual cycle. The menstrual cycle is typically 28 to 30 days long with the numbering system being the first day of menses counted as day one.

Days 1 through 7 are generally considered the period of menses where the levels of estrogen start to rise dramatically and progesterone level has already dropped off significantly. The lining of the uterus is sloughed off and the cycle begins anew.

Days 8 through 15 are concerned with selecting an egg (also called an ovum) and getting it ready for ovulation which occurs around day 14. During this time estrogen levels rise sharply and ovulation occurs with a spike of another hormone called Luteinizing Hormone or LH (which is the basis of the over-the-counter ovulation prediction kits sold in every pharmacy in the US).

Coincidentally, at the same time as ovulation a spike in the female levels of testosterone occurs. Testosterone is a known libido enhancer and I am certain that our species has been programmed to be especially receptive to sexual attraction around the time of ovulation.

The egg is ready for fertilization around day 14. The portion of the ovary responsible for that egg production is called the corpus luteum. This corpus luteum then begins to produce progesterone in large quantities in anticipation of a fertilized egg.

Days 15 - 22 or so result in a rapid and large increase in progesterone production. Once the body senses that the egg was not fertilized, then the progesterone component drops severely. The progesterone affects the lining of the uterus preparing it for a fertilized egg. The uterus gets enriched with blood vessels.

Once the progesterone level drops off, the overly enriched lining of the uterus sloughs off and the period begins anew, thus starting up the next cycle. A typical woman may have 400 cycles in her reproductive lifetime before this process gradually fades out into a menopausal state.

It is my observation that migraine headaches are the most common during the time that the progesterone levels rapidly fall off. This is the same time in the cycle that PMS symptoms are often present. PMS is associated with mood swings, excessive swelling, breast tenderness, decreased libido, weight gain, and in some women, migraine headaches.

My further observations of migraines in women include:

- ✓ the onset of headaches beginning with menarche (girls reaching puberty and beginning to have their first periods)

- ✓ onset or worsening of headaches with the administration of birth control pills.

- ✓ the relief or lessening of migraines during pregnancy

- ✓ the onset of headaches after the birth of the first child

- ✓ co-existence of migraines with depression

- ✓ correlation of migraines and post-partum depression – both due to crashing levels of progesterone

- ✓ the reduction of migraines in post-menopausal women

- ✓ the worsening or prolongation of migraines in post-menopausal women with the administration of (HRT) Premarin ® and other chemically-altered estrogens.

Now, **the really good news is that once we have figured what the real cause of migraines in women is, we know how to cure the problem**. Read on to find out what the cure is and how to make it work for YOU.

The Natural Hormones Dilemma –
Why Doctors Get Confused

It might be hard to believe, but most doctors are indeed confused about natural hormones and especially, progesterone. I was too at one time. Most doctors think a prescription drug called Provera® is the same thing as progesterone. It is not. Provera® is very different chemically.

The reason for this confusion is that we were taught in medical school that Provera® was progesterone. Generations of doctors have believed this and have no clue that Provera® is not progesterone. Furthermore, there is a progesterone-like (but again, not exactly progesterone) drug in birth control pills that doctors confuse with progesterone as well.

Well, here is why. This progesterone "look-alike" is actually a man-made product called Provera®. Provera® happens to be a so-called "progestin" that acts and has characteristics similar to progesterone, but it is NOT progesterone.

The drug company that manufactures Provera® actually takes the natural progesterone molecule and then ALTERS it by adding another chemical group to it. This chemical is another long chemical chain that when added to the base becomes the generic name: medroxy-progesterone. PROVERA® IS **NOT** PROGESTERONE.

All these classes of altered progesterone-like drugs are called progestins. This means that these progesterone look-alike drugs seem to resemble progesterone EXCEPT for some significant chemical alterations

37

which exert their effects on the human body. True, they do have some progesterone like effects BUT at the same time they have an enormous number of dangerous side effects.

Side effects of Provera® and other progestins in general were widely publicized in the renowned Women's Health Initiative study a few years ago that have blown the doors off of hormone replacement therapy. I have included a detailed description of this topic in my free report called *"What Nobody Told Women About Hormone Replacement Therapy"*.

The bottom line is that Provera ® and progestins have nasty side effects that include migraine headaches and cancer, just to name a few. The reason why this happens, in my observation, is that <u>these drugs poison the body's production of natural progesterone</u>, thus causing the deficiency of REAL progesterone and a relative imbalance of estrogen excess.

So, naturally comes a question - why do drug companies manufacture drugs that can potentially harm people? The existing patent laws are to blame. In this country and in most others, you cannot patent something that is already found in nature or is already natural. Therefore, in order to patent something, you HAVE to chemically change it into a non-natural substance. It is THAT simple.

This way, a drug company can then get a patent on this chemical and protect its costly research, development and testing investment in this drug. The reason why drug companies have to chemically alter progesterone into an artificial drug is because of the way that the patent laws are formulated. They just don't have a choice.

However, the problem is that once you alter a natural chemical found in the body into some other chemical that is "foreign" to the organism, that's when all of the side effects come into play.

A good example to show you how just a tiny alteration of a natural hormone can affect the body is the difference between estrogen and testosterone. These are both natural substances found in all humans, men and women. The only differences are the relative amounts of each, with women having a lot of estrogen and a little bit of testosterone and men with the exact opposite.

Looking at the chemical structures of estrogen and testosterone, they seem to be very similar. In fact, the only difference between these two hormones is a single double bond in one of the carbon rings.

Without having to go into complex and boring details from organic chemistry, I will say that the only difference between estrogen and testosterone is a single electron on an atomic level. It's that small and seemingly insignificant difference that separates the two main hormones that make a woman – a woman and a man – a man. Pretty impressive, isn't it?

If a single electron can thus produce the massive physiologic differences between men and women, imagine what an entire, long artificial chemical additive can do to an existing hormone! The side effects of these artificially altered hormones created to satisfy the requirements of the patent laws are tremendous and self-evident.

On the other hand, **natural hormones** (also called **bio-identical hormones**), like progesterone do not have these side effects and never will. The only effects that a natural product like progesterone can have are those that are dose-related and well known to human physiology. The reason is because in the case of NATURAL progesterone nothing chemically "foreign" is being introduced to the organism.

Of course, if you give someone a lot of progesterone, this will exert more progesterone effects than if you give a small amount of progesterone. It is so simple. These effects are well known and understood.

In fact, a "toxic" dose of progesterone is found in the human condition called - pregnancy!

The amount of the same natural progesterone that I supplement to my female patients is nowhere near the amounts of progesterone circulating in a pregnant woman's body. The amount of progesterone naturally produced by a pregnant woman can be a 100 fold higher than any amount that we could give you as a supplement.

Thus, unless the FDA and other countries' drug regulators begin labeling pregnancy as a dangerous condition, then we are extremely safe in administering natural progesterone to women.

Bio-identical progesterone is quite safe to take during pregnancy. In fact, we give it to enhance fertility and reduce the possibility of miscarriages. Bio-identical progesterone is routinely given during the first 10 weeks of pregnancy. After 10 weeks, a pregnant woman's elevated levels of progesterone overwhelm any supplemental dose that we give you.

Natural progesterone is quite safe to take while breast feeding. It is wonderful to eliminate post-partum depression which occurs when sky-high levels of circulating progesterone fall off a cliff after the baby is born. Progesterone deficiency, in addition to being a major cause of migraines, is also a cause of depression.

Finally, if all else fails, and a woman decides to go off supplemental progesterone, then she can just stop taking it – cold turkey. The body will wash it out over a few days and she returns back to her previous condition with no consequences.

The Wild Yam Goose Chase

There is a whole industry out there claiming that taking derivatives of wild yams will supplement the body with progesterone. A progesterone precursor, diosgenin, is found in abundance in wild yams. Numerous dietary supplement manufacturers' claim that the diosgenin found in their yams can supply the body with progesterone. Well, is that true?

"There is no evidence that the human body converts diosgenin (found in Mexican Wild Yam) to hormones", says Dr. David Zava (PhD in Bio Endocrinology whose focus has been progesterone and estrogen receptor activity), Laboratory Director of Aeron Life Cycles - one the foremost hormone testing facilities in the world.

Dr. Zava has tested progesterone levels for many thousands of women and responded with the following: "In response to your question about wild yam steroids - do they convert into progesterone? The answer is NO, there are no enzymes in the human body that will convert diosgenin, the active component of wild yams, into progesterone."

Don't waste your money on the "yam" supplements. They simply just don't work.

Migraines in Men

Now that the cause of migraines in women has been thoroughly developed, how do we account for migraines in men?

There is no definitive proof and we are extrapolating from women a similar theory for men. It was the sex hormones in women that were out of balance. The same should hold true for men. Fortunately, for men the sex hormones are much simpler. There are no fixed cycles to worry about and only one major hormone – TESTOSTERONE.

The severe headaches that men suffer are not as easily diagnosed as those in women. Men seem to experience two major types of debilitating headaches: migraines and cluster headaches.

The migraines that men experience are essentially identical to those that women have except for the monthly cycles which men don't have. These are easily diagnosed and probably do not occur as often as reported. The migraine headaches in women vastly outnumber those in men.

Cluster headaches are a different story. These are found almost exclusively in men. The intensity of this pain is so bad that suicide is a definite risk.

These are extremely painful, short bursts of headaches that last for minutes at a time, but can come in clusters over a period of a few hours. They are frequently night time headaches and can awaken someone from a sound sleep.

The pain from a cluster headache is also a little different with the description of ice pick type of pain associated with a myriad of vasomotor symptoms from the autonomic nervous system. The trigeminal nerve, carotid artery and tear ducts appear to play a large symptomatic role here.

Nevertheless, the literature discussing cluster headaches usually states that these headaches are distinctly different from migraines, but then acknowledge some overlapping similarities to migraines as well. Both, according to mainstream literature, suggest an association with serotonin levels.

As we have already learned from the women, anything connected with serotonin is also related to hormones in general. We have already noted a relationship with serotonin and the sex hormones in women and similar findings are found in men as well.

The primary sex hormone in men is testosterone. Therefore, my theory regarding migraine headaches and cluster headaches in men is that those are due to a deficiency of testosterone.

You ask, "Since when do men become deficient in testosterone?" Simple, like all other hormones, men and women peak at age 25 or so in the production of all hormones. After that, hormone production of all kinds declines about 1-3% per year thereafter.

Therefore, a 40 year old man will have 15-45% less testosterone than at age 25. How do you explain migraine headaches in a young man in his 20's? Again, if you look at the demographics of men with these types of headaches, especially, cluster headaches, many of them are overweight or obese.

In overweight/obese men fatty tissue acts in two ways. First, extra fatty tissue acts like a sponge and literally soaks up all kinds of circulating hormones thus lessening the amount available to the other organs in the body. Second, fatty tissue itself facilitates the conversion of testosterone to estrogen in some peripheral chemical reactions.

Just as women have an imbalance of progesterone with estrogen; men have an imbalance of testosterone with estrogen. The result is the same - with symptoms of severe headaches.

Migraine Treatment in Men

What are the dosages and route of administration for men with migraines?

The answer is to administer testosterone. Again, just like in the case of progesterone for women, testosterone is easiest to administer by mouth. Skin applications in a gel are available and there is an injectable version as well as an intra-muscular injection.

These are the recommended dosages:

Testosterone 50 mg, twice daily, by mouth. These are formulated by a compounding pharmacist.

Testosterone Cream 50 mg/gram. Apply ½ gram to skin twice daily.

Testosterone 100mg one time PER WEEK by IM injection.

Androgel comes in the form of a gel and is used at a rate of one packet per day applied to the skin. This is supposed to deliver 2.5 to 5 mg of testosterone per day.

There is one problem in all of the above testosterone recommendations: Because of recent political developments, Congress passed the Anabolic Steroids Act which basically criminalized possession of testosterone and converted it into what is called a Schedule III drug.

This places testosterone and most other anabolic hormone substances into the same political class as narcotics. Possession without a prescription is a crime (felony). Therefore, all of the above recommended testosterone administrations are perfectly legal, but they MUST be prescribed by a doctor who is comfortable with prescribing Schedule III drugs.

In the event that a man cannot obtain testosterone, a backup recommendation is to take DHEA, a precursor to testosterone.

The recommended dose for DHEA, in the absence of testosterone administration is between 200mg and 400mg of DHEA per day.

THE CURE: How To SUCCESSFULLY Treat Migraines

Before I begin, many of you are so motivated that you just read the table of contents and skip immediately to this section and start reading from here.

Because there is quite a bit of background building up to this section, I recommend you start from the beginning. The first 28 pages are relatively easy to read and should only take about 30 minutes of your time. Or you can start here, but do go back later and read from the beginning.

WAIT!

Even if you read nothing else on this page – **I urge you to at least carefully go over the critical information found below** - it's that important!

The Following Information Is

VITALLY IMPORTANT TO YOUR HEALTH

You may be anxious about **"hormones"** – many people are. We've heard so much sensationalized news lately about hormone abuse, it's sometimes difficult to separate **fact from fiction**.

Here's the straight story:

- **Migraines are largely caused by a sex hormone deficiency**, though other factors can also play a role.

- **Birth control pills and standard hormone replacement therapy (HRT) are <u>not</u> natural.** They contain chemical "mimics" that only approximate your natural hormones. These mimics are not only **harmful to your body**, but actually cause you to stop making your own NATURAL sex hormones.

- We **<u>make migraine headaches go away</u>** by replenishing deficiencies in your **natural** hormone levels.

- **We use only natural, bio-identical hormones** to replace the deficient hormones your body is lacking.

- Bio-identical hormones are **VERY DIFFERENT** from the hormones you read about in the newspaper. The **prescription hormones** you may have taken in the past (either as birth control pills or HRT) **are NOT NATURAL.**

- **Synthetic hormones are foreign chemicals, acting as poisons.** They shut down your ovaries. They do cause cancer as well as many other health problems.

- However, **<u>BIO-IDENTICAL HORMONES ARE TOTALLY NATURAL!</u>** They are EXACTLY THE SAME as the hormones produced in your own body. **They are absolutely safe** and cannot harm you. They do not cause or contribute to cancer.

- **Mother Nature** would never make a harmful natural hormone. If natural or bio-identical hormones **were** harmful, why don't we see cancers and other health problems in 25 year olds, when hormone production peaks? We don't.

> - People get health problems when they take **synthetic, chemically altered hormones** that **interfere with the body's production of natural hormones**, or when their natural hormone levels decline.

Mainstream Medicine Fails

There is the mainstream medicine method of treating migraine headaches which is addressing the symptoms only, and then there is my way – which is **the curative, preventative way**.

First, you should be thoroughly familiar with the mainstream method. If you have downloaded this e-book, then chances are you have already tried NSAIDS (anti-inflammatory medications), anti-depressants, "triptans" (Amerge®, Maxalt®, Imitrex®, Avert®, Frova®, Zomig®, Relpax®), and possibly even DHE (dihydroergotamine), or all of the above.

In 2006, estimated sales of the triptans alone are expected to be nearly US$4 billion. Imitrex® (made by Glaxo Smith Kline) has the largest share of the triptan market accounting for about US$1.2 billion in sales alone.

The drug companies have found a partial short term solution to the problem, and have developed these drugs to accommodate a desperate population. Many migraine sufferers do not mind (or have no other choice) paying some US$73 for a two-dose shot of Imitrex®.

Virtually all of the major drug companies now have their own proprietary triptan drug out on the market and they want you to take their version. They have a lot of money invested in these products. It costs hundreds of millions of dollars to research, develop, and pass it through the FDA study process before they get FDA approval to take it to market.

The last thing a drug company needs is to find out that somebody out there has found a cure to the problem that they are making billions off of. Two bad things happen to the drug company at that point:

a) They won't be able to sell any more US$73 doses of medications.
b) They just lost several hundred million dollars in development costs.

Therefore, the big drug companies, in partnership with the FDA, will do everything possible to shut down any "natural" source or cure for ANY medical condition that they have invested their money in because natural cures are bad for their business. This also happens to include migraine headaches. And this means that YOU, the migraine sufferer, will be intentionally denied information and access to any natural, non-prescription or curative product that will make the big drug companies' drugs obsolete.

I will spare you the detailed discussion of these medications. Most of you have already taken one or more of these medications already.

If these medications had worked so well, you would not be reading this book right now. So, assuming that this is correct, then you are ready for the definitive cure for your migraine headaches. I say "definitive" because about 80% of people that I treat are indeed cured by this method.

Why only 80%? Why not 100%?

As with any complicated medical problem we are not always correct in our diagnosis or complete understanding of the underlying disease process. Perhaps the other 20% have some other variation of headache that we are labeling a migraine but is actually something quite different? And a certain percentage of these people just don't respond as well as we would like to our usual hormone treatment.

If either the progesterone deficiency theory or the estrogen excess withdrawal theory is correct, then the supplementation of progesterone will almost always correct the condition.

This is why curing migraines is so simple and easy – all we do is just add back to women enough progesterone to correct the deficiency in progesterone. We also try to correct the nutritional deficiencies in magnesium, iodine and Vitamin D as adjuncts to progesterone therapy.

Similarly we would do the same thing for men by adding back testosterone that they are deficient in. Men are equally deficient in the other nutrients, as well.

This is also why it is 100% natural. Progesterone that is manufactured to exactly match the chemical structure of the real hormone that circulates throughout your body is called **bio-identical**. This is a **natural**

substance that every one of us has because our bodies manufacture it on a daily basis.

Please note that I will use the terms "bio-identical hormone" and "natural hormone" interchangeably. They mean exactly the same thing.

To supplement someone with more progesterone that is bio-identical is to do so utilizing an entirely natural approach. All we are doing is supplying in enough quantity to satisfy what the body truly needs to function better.

The results are so striking and occur so quickly that it is gratifying to watch the results.

Women get a little more complicated because we have to deal with the menstrual cycle and get the timing just right within the cycle. Menstruating females ideally will be taking progesterone immediately after ovulation has occurred.

Thus menstruating women should take progesterone supplementation during days 15 -28 (or 30) of their cycle. It may take a couple of cycles or so for the migraines (and other gynecological problems) to go away.

A menstruating woman could theoretically take progesterone every day, but this is not usually done when a woman is trying to get pregnant. There is no harm in taking progesterone every day for a menstruating woman, however.

Specifically, progesterone taken during the first half of the menstrual cycle tends to decrease the production of mucous secreted by the uterus. Mucous helps the sperm swim toward the awaiting egg during ovulation.

Also progesterone taken in high dosages can actually suppress ovulation. (This is why pregnant women don't ovulate. – Think about that situation!). But we have many menstruating women taking progesterone on a daily basis for differing reasons. See the comments when I go over the dosage requirements later in this book.

Independent of migraine headaches, for those women who are actively trying to get pregnant, we routinely add progesterone in the second half of the cycle to encourage fertilized egg implantation. Progesterone also prevents or lowers the incidence of miscarriage in the early portion of pregnancy.

Therefore progesterone is quite safe to take for any woman whether they want to get pregnant or not.

Nevertheless, as a matter of routine, we do not usually start out taking progesterone in the first half of your cycle if you are still having periods.

For post-menopausal women, it is much simpler. Take progesterone every single day. No worries, no stress. Very simple. Results come quickly.

What if you are peri-menopausal?

For those of you who do not fall into the traditional classifications of having regular periods (normal menstruating women) and those having no periods (post menopausal) many of you will fall into the "peri-menopausal" group of being in between.

The peri-menopausal woman is typically in her early to late 40's. She is still having periods, but becoming more irregular. The periods can either get lighter and shorter or longer and heavier.

Those peri-menopausal women whose periods are getting longer and heavier typically have uterine fibroids and have been told they may need a hysterectomy. Many have already had a hysterectomy.

For purposes of discussing migraine headache treatment with progesterone, we separate out those who desire to get pregnant from those who do not. Peri-menopausal women, by definition are pretty much out of the pregnancy running.

So we treat peri-menopausal women as a post-menopausal woman when it comes to hormone replacement with natural progesterone. Alternatively, if you are 37 years old, still cycling normally, but no longer desire to get pregnant, you can take your progesterone supplementation just like the post-menopausal women. There are certain advantages to this schedule as you will see later when we start talking about dosing schedules.

Once the hysterectomy issue comes up, then we get into new categories: those who had a hysterectomy and kept the ovaries and those whose ovaries were removed with the hysterectomy.

Frankly, it doesn't matter whether you have had a hysterectomy or not. Your hormones are still circulating around and every cell in your body is still being affected by them, whether you have a uterus or not.

If your ovaries have been removed, then you discovered a condition called "surgical menopause". This means that while you were still recovering in the hospital following your surgery, you felt immediate menopausal symptoms of hot flashes and night sweats. Because of the sudden shock to your body, this was an intense condition and is likely still troubling you.

I do not intend to go into any detail about menopausal symptoms. We will save that for future topics, but for now as far as progesterone supplementation is concerned, your body is doubly short of progesterone. (By the way, an excellent information website on menopause is www.1-Menopause.com).

Your ovaries are the primary manufacturer of your progesterone and estrogen. When the ovaries were removed your body went into hormone shock. But your body's cells still need those hormones.

The good news is that your adrenal glands can manufacture hormones including progesterone and estrogen. The bad news is that they can't put out the same quantities that your ovaries could make.

The bottom line on natural progesterone supplementation for those of you with hysterectomies, with or without ovarian removal, is that you are now out of the pregnancy class and into the menopausal class. This means you take progesterone supplements every day.

What if you are taking birth control pills?

There is one major step that women **must** do before we start correcting any progesterone deficiency – and that is to **stop taking any birth control pills immediately.** I cannot stress how important it is to discontinue oral contraceptives.

If you do not stop taking birth control pills, then it does not matter what we do, or how much progesterone we give you, you will not get better. Find another method of birth control, just get off the pills. This is not a suggestion, it is mandatory. **Birth control pills are a MAJOR reason why you are getting migraines** if you are a woman.

Stopping birth control pills is not just limited to the oral pills. The same toxic synthetic, chemically altered hormones are also found in birth control patches (Ortho-Evra) and implants like Norplant as well as IUD's and must be removed, as well.

Occasionally, some women say that they cannot get off birth control pills for a variety of legitimate reasons. Under those circumstances where stopping birth control pills is not an option, then we do have a strategy in place to deal with this.

It is called, "Match the Pill" strategy whereby we simply add a natural progesterone every day that a birth control pill is taken. For further information, the following website is a good source: www.DitchThePill.org .

Synthetic hormone replacement drugs like PremPro must also be discontinued. There is more discussion on PremPro later, but this drug gets included in the same category as birth control pills as it is virtually identical to them.

In a nutshell, the reason why birth control pills are so bad for you is because they poison and shut down the body's production of natural progesterone by the ovaries. They also saturate the bloodstream with extra estrogen, giving the worst case scenario of excessive estrogen and insufficient progesterone at the same time.

Please refer to my Special Report, *What Nobody Told Women About Birth Control Pills* for more detailed information on birth control pills and how they have poisoned women across the world.

Now, read on for more details on dosages and exactly what to do and where to get it.

The Secret Mineral that Will Boost the Effectiveness of Your Program and What No Pharmacist Will Tell You about It

So, what's that magic mineral that makes the sex hormone supplementation program of treating migraine headaches even more effective and what's so secret about it? Well, believe it or not, it's good old magnesium. Why? The importance of magnesium for the human body cannot be underestimated. Magnesium is used in over two hundred chemical reactions in a human body.

What's The Secret? Take This and Get an Even Better Response

Magnesium can act synergistically with progesterone to help suppress migraines. There have been two fairly good studies showing that women with migraines tend to be deficient in ionized magnesium. One study showed that 45% of women with migraines were low in magnesium.

Keep in mind that about a fourth of the general population is also deficient in magnesium. So there appears to be a higher incidence of magnesium deficiency in women with migraines.

One study demonstrated a reduction in migraine attacks with the administration of intravenous magnesium. Another study demonstrated a reduction in migraines taking oral magnesium during the last 15 days of the menstrual cycle.

Our clinic has noticed that if you combine magnesium with progesterone supplementation, migraine headaches resolve more quickly than just taking the progesterone alone.

Therefore, we always recommend taking magnesium. But the magnesium has to be a special type that is a little harder to find and that is precisely the "secret" part. There is somewhat of a long explanation to this as people just assume that "magnesium is just magnesium".

Not so.

Please bear with me as it is rather important to explain why getting the right type of magnesium is necessary if we want magnesium to help and give our progesterone supplementation a boost in effectiveness.

Magnesium taken in the form of magnesium oxide is the most common preparation on store and pharmacy shelves. There is a reason for that: It is cheaper to manufacture and comes in a high quantity for the size of the pill.

The problem with magnesium oxide is that it is absorbed and filtered out of the body in about an hour. If you try to take it more often, you get diarrhea – not a pleasant long term solution.

So we recommend taking magnesium in the form of a compound that ends with an "ate". Chemical compounds that end in an "ate" are called "chelates".

Chelates are nature's way of neutralizing chemically charged molecules. Magnesium, all by itself, is a mineral that carries an electric charge. It is kind of like a battery. But your body does not like electrically charged substances without some insulation.

So magnesium chelates act as insulators by binding up a molecule that carries that exact opposite electric charge of magnesium. Place the magnesium with the chelate and presto, you have a neutral, zero charged chemical complex.

A magnesium chelate vastly improves the body's ability to absorb and take it up for immediate use in the myriad of physiological reactions where it is required.

The following are all examples of magnesium chelates.

- Magnesium aspartate,
- Magnesium gluconate,
- Magnesium glycinate,
- Magnesium stearate,
- And/or magnesium citrate

These are the best magnesium supplements to take because they absorb the best, last longer inside the body and are cleared more slowly by the kidneys.

However, each of the magnesium chelate compounds will last inside the body for a particular time, like 2 hours to 8 hours. They all have different "peaks" and "valleys" in terms of how much magnesium is released inside the body.

The idea is to find a magnesium supplement that combines multiple chelates into one pill so your body can have continuous high magnesium coverage for up to eight hours. Then you take this ideal magnesium pill just three times a day and you are covered with sufficient magnesium.

We found one magnesium product that actually contains not one, but three of the above magnesium chelates. This will be described for you in the "How Do We Get These Treatments" chapter later in this book. I will also tell you how you can get your own magnesium chelate formula as one of your treatment options.

Neptune Krill Oil – Nature's Remedy from the Sea

Neptune Krill Oil (NKO) is a remarkable new product that features a natural turbo-charged omega-3 fish oil. One particular type of Krill oil called Neptune Krill Oil has specially integrated omega-3 essential fatty acids – EPA and DHA - that are three times more easily absorbed by the body.

The resulting product is like a supercharged fish oil that is one of the most powerful anti-oxidants on the planet and a very potent anti-inflammatory agent. Yet it is entirely natural, contains no dangerous heavy metals or pesticides and has no fishy aftertaste.

What is unique about Neptune Krill Oil is two-fold: location of where the krill comes from and the process by which it is formulated.

Krill are small shrimp-like crustaceans that inhabit the oceans in very cold, deep water off of Antarctica. They are a major food supply for whales, squid, fish and seals. Krill are also found near the Arctic, as well, but they are not as pure as the Antarctic variety.

Neptune is a unique formulation keeping the purity of the krill intact while adding a powerful anti-oxidant to an already potent, naturally occurring substance. It is clearly superior to "generic" brands.

The omega-3 fatty acids in Neptune Krill Oil are exclusively EPA and DHA, which come in the form of phospholipids contrary to all other marine oils where the fatty acids are in a triglyceride form. What this means is that the NKO is significantly more bioavailable than fish oil because it allows for direct absorption of EPA and DHA across cell membranes.

The ratio is about 3 to 1, with NKO being absorbed three times faster than traditional fish oil. It passes through the stomach and small intestine so fast that the chance for a fishy aftertaste or reflux is virtually eliminated.

Antioxidant Benefits of Neptune Krill Oil

What makes Neptune Krill Oil so beneficial? It has already been measured to be a very powerful anti-oxidant. Using the Oxygen Radical Absorbance Capacity (ORAC) studies which measure the strength of antioxidant power, NKO has a value 300 times higher than vitamin E and 35 times more potent than Coenzyme Q10. NKO is 47 times more potent as an anti-oxidant than standard fish oil.

Anti-inflammatory Benefits of Neptune Krill Oil

A study showed that Neptune Krill Oil can significantly reduce inflammation by lowering C-reactive protein (CRP) by 30.9% after taking 300mg/day for a period of 30 days. C-reactive protein is one of the most important markers of inflammation measured in blood studies.

Neptune Krill Oil and PMS

A study performed at the University of Montreal and published in the May, 2003 issue of the Alternative Medicine Review, demonstrated a statistically significant improvement in PMS symptoms as measured by a Self-Assessment Questionnaire for the

American College of Obstetricians and Gynecologists (ACOG) diagnostic criteria for PMS.

Seventy women took Neptune Krill Oil for 45 days, 90 days or three cycles and demonstrated improvement versus baseline groups who simply took fish oil alone.

This same study also revealed a significant reduction in pain medications needed for dysmenorrheal (painful periods) by those women who took NKO.

Neptune Krill Oil is Synergistic with other Treatments

We have found that the combination of natural progesterone with Neptune Krill Oil and multi-chelated magnesium (see next chapter for magnesium discussion) results in an improvement with overall treatment of migraines.

Obviously, the biggest component is the natural progesterone. Bio-identical progesterone alone works pretty well. Then we added the magnesium product which helped even more.

But the addition of the Neptune Krill Oil seems to be another accomplishment to the treatment recommendations. We have raised our success rates even higher with this combination. It gets even better when we add iodine and Vitamin D. More on that later.

Iodine – The "Back Door" to Your Thyroid

One thing we have learned within the last year is that iodine is critical. This edition of this book is including my blanket recommendation for iodine supplementation.

Why? Because almost everyone on the planet doesn't have enough iodine in their thyroid gland, much less in their body. This means that almost everyone is at risk of an under-active thyroid (hypothyroidism).

Most Women with Migraines have Low Thyroid

I have found that many, if not most, women with migraine headaches have low thyroid. In the past, we would write a prescription for thyroid hormone which has its own set of risks - and problems finding the right dosage. Of course, most mainstream doctors refuse to write a prescription for thyroid hormone in the face of "normal" thyroid blood tests.

The following are some of the major symptoms and signs associated with an under-active thyroid:

- Depression
- Weight gain
- Difficulty losing weight
- Low energy - fatigue
- Cold natured
- Ice-cold hands or feet
- Dry skin
- Hair loss (alopecia)
- Slowed thinking, poor concentration
- Brain fog

- Memory problems
- Insomnia, poor sleep
- Waking up exhausted
- Tingling in hands and feet
- Muscle pain
- Edema (swelling in ankles)
- Constipation
- Slow heart rate
- Low blood pressure
- Elevated cholesterol
- Thickened tongue
- Anemia
- Thinned eyebrows
- Slow reflexes
- Cool body temperature

With simple iodine replacement, we can make the symptoms of an under active thyroid go away much of the time without ever having to prescribe thyroid hormone!

Iodine replacement is safe, cheap and effective. And it does much more than fix your thyroid. More on that later...

I must give credit to two giant pioneers in this field: Dr. David Brownstein and Dr. Guy Abraham. Dr. Brownstein has a wonderful book on Iodine, now in its 3rd edition that you can read, called *Iodine – Why You Need It – Why YouCan't Live without It.* Much of my information is derived from his book and his lecture to the International Hormone Society in March of 2008, which I attended.

You can order the book from his website:
http://www.drbrownstein.com

Iodine Deficiency is Epidemic

In a study of 4000 patients with Dr. Brownstein, 96% of them were found to be deficient in iodine. According to the World Health Organization, 72% of the world's population is affected by iodine deficiency.

This trend is worsening. Over the last 30 years, the NHANES (National Health and Nutrition Examination Survey I) shows that iodine levels have dropped 50% (in the U.S.).

Why Are People Iodine Deficient?

There is a double reason for iodine deficiencies: inadequate intake and exposure to toxicities that displace iodine.

Iodine is a mineral. It is not abundant in the earth. Iodine is found primarily in seawater and in very small quantities and in soils near the ocean. Soils are naturally deficient in iodine, especially the further away or inland you get from the ocean.

Iodine is also fairly easily displaced from your body by toxins called toxic halides.

Along with iodine, other common halides are fluoride, bromine and chlorine. Fluoride is found in toothpaste and in your water supply. Bromine is found in bakery products, breads, pastas, swimming pool chemicals and a number of medicines. Chlorine is found in many chemical residues ranging from pesticides (dioxin) and thousands of other man-made chemicals.

The water supply is bad. Every time you take a shower or drink from the tap, your body gets a little exposure to fluoride, which leeches out good iodine.

Why is Iodine Important?

I was taught in medical school that the thyroid gland was the ONLY organ that uses iodine. How wrong!!

Yes, iodine is critical for the function of thyroid hormone production. And we will dwell on this further. But there was (and remains today incredible ignorance by the medical schools regarding teaching on any other body function regarding iodine).

Iodine is present and is used in every single cell in your body, including your eyeballs and retina.

The thyroid gland does contain more iodine than any other organ (barely – breast tissue uses almost as much iodine).

But large amounts of iodine are stored in:

- Salivary glands
- CSF and the brain
- Gastric mucosa
- Choroid plexus (part of the brain)
- Breasts
- Ovaries
- Eye – ciliary bodies

Mainstream medicine even concedes that iodine deficiency can result in ADD, mental retardation (cretinism), deafness (also a part of cretinism), goiter, increased infant and child mortality, infertility. Iodine deficiency is the most common preventable form of mental retardation known.

Iodine Storage Needs

Your body should store a minimum of 6 mg/day of iodine in your thyroid gland and 5 mg/day in your breast tissue (if you are female).

Total daily iodine storage needs for your body (female) are about 12 -13 mg/day of iodine (minimum). Note that US RDA levels for iodine are 150 mcg/day. That is 150 MICROgrams and we just noted that the body actually needs about 12 or 13 MILLIgrams. One milligram = 1000 micrograms.

Do the math and the RDA figures are about 100 times less than what modern science shows we really need.

Where Does Iodine Come From?

We already know that the soil and therefore, the food supply, is deficient in iodine. Except for the Japanese who consume large amounts of kelp seaweed, it can be assumed that everyone else does not get sufficient iodine from the diet.

Your next question is "We have iodized salt. Isn't that sufficient?" Answer: No.

Some may think that iodization of salt has eliminated iodine deficiency. Not true. Iodized salt only has 10%

bioavailability. Also note that less than 50% of the population even uses iodized salt. We have been programmed for many years to avoid salt in our diets. Even so, it would not be sufficient.

From 1960 until 1980, iodine was added to bakery items. But one erroneous study stirred fears of iodine toxicity, so in 1980 iodine was replaced with bromine. Bad move.

Now with the addition of bromine to bakery items, not only did we lose a significant source of iodine but it was replaced with a toxin that actually leeches iodine from your body.

The good news is that the process works the other way around. Supplementation of iodine actually removes toxic halides (bromine, fluoride and chlorine) from your body.

Iodine and the Thyroid Gland:

There are actually four types of thyroid hormones. The four hormones are determined by the number of iodine molecules in them. They are designated as T1, T2, T3, and T4. The most important are T3 and T4.

T4 is called thyroxin and has four iodine molecules. T3 is called tri-iodothyronine and has three iodine molecules. T3 is only the biologically active thyroid hormone.

The bottom line is that if there is not enough iodine in the thyroid gland, then it is impossible to have sufficient thyroid hormone of any type resulting in under active thyroid or hypothyroidism.

I will write about the thyroid in more detail in my chapter "What To Do if All Else Fails (The 20%)?" later in this book.

As recently as 2007, progressive doctors such as me, wrote prescriptions for thyroid hormones in patients who clinically manifested hypothyroid symptoms (regardless of blood tests). And this was relatively successful.

Now, we are finding out that iodine supplementation alone helps half (or more) of our patients without ever having to resort to the prescription pad and hassle of getting a doctor to write a script for thyroid hormone.

This is win-win situation.

Types of Iodine:

There are two types of iodine: Iodine and iodide. One is a reduced form, meaning that there is an extra electron.

I don't want to spend too much time discussing chemistry but the bottom line is that Dr. Brownstein and Dr. Abraham have extensive research showing that it requires both forms of iodine and iodide for optimal bioavailability.

Iodine Supplementation

Per Dr. Brownstein, the current recommendation for iodine supplementation is a minimum of 12.5 mg of an iodine/iodide combination per day. The maximum recommended dose is 150 mg of the iodine/iodide combination per day. This is 100 times the outdated US RDA recommendations.

Moderate iodine deficiencies will require 25 – 50 mg/day. For people with thyroid antibodies, they should take 50 mg/day.

Dr. G. Abraham's research shows that by adding Vitamin B2 (riboflavin) and Vitamin B3 (niacin), this helps maximize the effect of iodine supplementation. In fact, by adding the B2 and B3 you can probably just get away with taking the minimal iodine/iodide dosage (12.5 mg) and do just fine.

Selenium

Selenium is necessary for proper functioning of the enzyme, iodothyronine deiodinase. This is the enzyme that is critical for conversion of T4 into T3 (the active thyroid hormone).

Selenium is recommended to enhance the conversion of T4 into T3. With supplementation of selenium, you can achieve higher levels of active thyroid hormone.

The maximum daily dose of selenium should not exceed 400 mg/day.

Iodine and Migraines

So why is iodine important for migraine sufferers? Because most migaineurs have varying low thyroid levels and we believe that this is largely a result of insufficient iodine.

In our experience, basically anything that enhances thyroid function, whether we prescribe thyroid hormone directly or take iodine supplements that boost thyroid function, the end result is better.

Obviously, supplementing with progesterone is still the primary treatment modality for women with migraines, but enhancing thyroid function does improve our results and is just a better overall quality of life.

Recommendations

12.5 mg/day of an iodine/iodide combination plus Vitamin B2, Vitamin B3 and Selenium.

50 mg/day of the above combination for people with thyroid auto-antibodies.

Source: www.IodinePlus.com

Vitamin D – "Vitamin of the Year"

One of my new recommendations for 2008 is the supplementation with Vitamin D. At a recent conference in Las Vegas hosted by the International Hormone Society, one of the lecturers called Vitamin D, "The vitamin of the year".

To summarize why: Practically everyone on the planet is deficient in Vitamin D (much to the dismay of academia). The other thing we are finding out is just how important Vitamin D really is.

If you thought (as I was taught in medical school) that Vitamin D is just good for keeping your bones strong, then you will be shocked at the vast number of functions of Vitamin D.

If you thought (as I was taught in medical school) that all you need is a few minutes of sunshine to get sufficient vitamin D for the day, then you are terribly mistaken.

We are in a new world. Vitamin D is much more important than we previously believed and EVERYONE IS DEFICIENT in Vitamin D.

Who is Vitamin D Deficient?

Dr. Damien Downing, President of the *British Society for Ecological Medicine*, says we ALL are.

The Mayo Clinic says that "overall 93% of 150 schoolchildren and adults" were deficient in Vitamin D in a Minnesota-based study. Within that study, the Mayo Clinic found that 100% of African Americans,

East Africans, Hispanics and American Indians were deficient.

The New England Journal of Medicine as far back as the March 19, 1998 issue had a headline saying, "Vitamin D Deficiency is Pandemic".

If you think sunlight helps, think again. The journal, *Spine*, in 2003 stated that 83% of people that were studied with chronic back pain in Saudi Arabia were vitamin D deficient.

The Science of Vitamin D

Before I go on, there is more than one version of Vitamin D. I am referring to the active form known as D3 or cholecalciferol. The terms "Vitamin D" and "D3" can be used interchangeably. There is a D2 version, but it is inactive and must be converted into D3 before it has any effects on the human body.

The science of Vitamin D has exploded in the last few years. But careful review of the literature hints of the importance of Vitamin D. Only recently has the enormity of the role that Vitamin D been revealed in one blockbuster study after another.

Inflammation:

We are just beginning to scratch the surface regarding the study of inflammation. What is inflammation? Basically the body is inflamed or stressed. Long term this can lead to chronic diseases like lupus, rheumatoid arthritis, inflammatory bowel disease (ulcerative colitis and Crohn's Disease), chronic pain, muscle pain, heart disease, depression, dementia and especially cancers.

NF-kappaB

So inflammation is important. One of the major recent findings on inflammation was the discovery of NF-kappaB. This NF-kappaB lives in the cytosol of cells and appears to be the major promoter of the inflammatory pathway. It is activated by injury, radiation, stress, allergens, viral infections, certain prostaglandins, toxins (like pesticides), low levels of omega fatty acids and, you guessed it, low levels of Vitamin D.

Basically anything bad promotes inflammation. Vitamin D deficiency and inflammation was confirmed recently as correlated with heart failure in the Jan 5, 2008, issue of the *Journal American Geriatric Society*.

Vitamin D's influence on down-regulating NF-kappaB was more recently described in the March, 2007 issue of *Journal of Steroid Biochemistry and Molecular Biology*.

But as early as 1995, similar science described Vitamin D's role in down regulating NF-kappaB in the journal *Immunology, Proceedings of the National Academy of Science*.

Cancers and More

I attended a lecture in May of 2008 in Vancouver at the *International Conference of Orthomolecular Medicine* where Dr. Damien Downing, MB, author of the book, *"Day Light Robbery"*, which describes Vitamin D deficiency and function, states that we are ALL deficient in Vitamin D.

He makes some interesting observations:

- 11 kinds of cancer are correlated with Vitamin D deficiency.

- Most cancer cells have increased numbers of Vitamin D receptors, so they may be plausibly more susceptible to Vitamin D effects.

- Vitamin D is a potent inhibitor of tumor cell induced angiogenesis (meaning that Vitamin D can make cancer cells lose their blood supply and ability to expand).

- Vitamin D strikingly inhibits cell proliferation and induces cell apoptosis (inability to divide) in breast cancer, prostate cancer and osteosarcoma.

- Influenza epidemics are correlated with Vitamin D deficiency.

- Vitamin D is lower in obese people.

- Vitamin D suppresses leptins (which are correlated with obesity)

Why are We Deficient in Vitamin D?

Dr. Downing says that there is a worldwide deficiency in Vitamin D for three reasons:

- Lack of sunlight
- Dietary deficiency
- Farming practices

Studies, new and old demonstrate a worldwide deficiency of Vitamin D in just about everyone. Living in sun-drenched areas does not help. We knew for some time that living north of the tropics was a problem. But the study from Saudi Arabia opened some eyes as to the real extent of Vitamin D deficiency.

The New England Journal of Medicine was right when it said we are in a "Vitamin D Deficiency Pandemic".

We now know the importance of diet to all essential ingredients, not just Vitamin D. Worldwide, diets are increasingly deficient in just about all good nutrients. Thousands of years of farming have depleted soils. Animal sources are depleted.

The myths of over supplementation with Vitamin D are largely debunked. Supplementation with Vitamin D in very high doses is safe and necessary.

Vitamin D and Migraines:

Where does Vitamin D fit in with treatment for migraine headaches? There is no specific research on Vitamin D with migraines. However, in the last year we have basically starting putting everyone on Vitamin D supplements whether they have migraines or not. We are seeing some anecdotal improvement in the migraines but mainly people are just feeling a little better overall.

I think the general health issue is important when we try to treat specific conditions such as migraines. We can try to correct hormone deficiencies all we want, but if the general condition of the patient is not good or more aptly described as "inflammatory" then it makes sense to treat the whole person.

In the face of near universal deficiency, I have now added the crucial supplement of Vitamin D to our migraine regimen. Take 5000 IU/day.

While you are at it, put your whole family on Vitamin D. We all need it.

Dosages

Another lecture presented in Houston by Dr. Abbas Qutab in September, 2007, recommended Vitamin D supplementation to be 4000 IU/day, up from 400 IU the previous RDA levels.

The journal *Steroids*, recommended 50,000 – 100,000 IU/week combined with calcium (1500mg) which resulted in normalization of menstrual periods.

It seems that the recommended supplementation levels for Vitamin D have increased more than 10 fold since the original RDA levels decades ago. New science has revealed the sweeping multiple functions of Vitamin D way above and beyond anything that mainstream doctors were taught.

The latest recommendation is 5000 IU/day.

THE PLAN: Exact Dosages and Administration

Print this section out and read it carefully.

Be sure and read every word in this section, even in those sections that you don't think apply to you because some of the comments apply to all women, regardless of category.

After years of practice, a lot of trial and error, and incredible feedback from my early patients who were not afraid of some experimentation, we have finally figured out the best overall doses of progesterone to give.

CATEGORY #1:
For Menstruating Women:

Be sure and know which category you are in. There is a detailed discussion in the "How Do We Treat Migraines" section above describing who is considered to be a menstruating woman and who is not in the category (even if you are still having periods).

The best rule of thumb is that if you are having periods and are of child bearing age and still desire (or would not mind) having any more children, then you are considered to be in the menstruating woman category.

The age group for this category begins with young girls experiencing their very first periods up to women approaching age 40. We have successfully treated girls as young as 13 who were going through menarche, which is the medical term given for having your very first periods.

1. The best dose to give a menstruating woman (Category 1) is 50 mg of bio-identical or natural progesterone given twice daily from days 15 until your period starts (for most women this is around day 28 – 30).

2. In addition to the progesterone recommended dosage, to make this treatment plan work even better, take 100 mg of long-acting magnesium, three times a day, EVERY DAY.

3. Take Krill Oil, a superior form of omega-3 fatty acids, one gel cap twice daily. EVERY DAY.

4. Take a minimum of 12.5 mg of Iodine daily. EVERY DAY.

5. Take 5000 IU of Vitamin D3 daily. EVERY DAY.

If you are currently taking birth control pills, do not start taking the bio-identical progesterone until you finish out your last round of birth control pills. In other words, regardless of where you are on the birth control pack, finish all 28 pills (or 21 if your pack comes this way) and wait for your menstrual period to start as usual. Then you can throw away your remaining oral contraceptives forever.

A special note on young girls and teenagers who are experiencing terrible periods and have migraine headaches: Almost all of them have been placed on birth control pills by mainstream medicine and this just worsens the migraines. So your daughters who are caught in this situation need to get off the pill as described in the preceding paragraph.

Remember that day one of your cycle is the first day of bleeding with your period. So after you finish your birth control pills for the prior month, then begin with the progesterone on day 15 of the following month. Then continue to take as instructed above – from day 15 until your period starts. For many women this is day 28, others day 30. The exact day is not important. Just continue to take it until bleeding begins. Then you can start back on the next day 15.

If you are not taking oral contraceptives currently, you can just start taking the progesterone the next time your day 15 comes up. Timing is very important, so you don't want to jump the gun and start taking these bio-identical progesterone hormones too soon or too late.

CATEGORY #2:
For The Following Groups:

- **Non-Menstruating** *or*
- **Post Menopausal Women** *or*
- **Peri-Menopausal** *or*
- **Women with Hysterectomies** *or*
- **Women who no longer desire children:**

This category is for everybody else. For classification purposes we will call this giant category the "Post-Menopausal Category". There will be discussion below on post-menopausal dosage changes and all of the women who are peri-menopausal and those with hysterectomies will be considered to be part of this post-menopausal group.

We can even include those of you who are not yet peri-menopausal, are somewhere around your late 30's and desire no more children.

This category is much simpler because we don't have to count days anymore.

1. The best dose to give a Category 2 woman is 50 mg of bio-identical or natural progesterone given twice daily, EVERY DAY.

2. In addition to the progesterone recommended dosage, to make this treatment plan work even better, take 100 mg of long-acting magnesium, three times a day, EVERY DAY.

3. Take Krill Oil, a superior form of omega-3 fatty acids, one gel cap twice daily. EVERY DAY.

4. Take a minimum of 12.5 mg of Iodine daily. EVERY DAY.

5. Take 5000 IU of Vitamin D3 daily. EVERY DAY.

Notice that the 5 recommendations are identical to those for menstruating women (category 1), except for the progesterone, which is taken every day for the second major category.

There is no need to have a periodic week off (literally). Natural progesterone is so safe that you can take it every day, forever.

At the recommended dosages your periods, if any, are not likely to change much. If they do change, they will get lighter, shorter or disappear altogether. This is not a problem and we have never had any woman complain about lighter, shorter or no periods.

Range of Dosages:

Smaller doses are helpful, but these dosages are usually not curative. Higher doses are safe as well, but we don't want to start out too high. This is the Goldilocks principle – not too small, not too large, but just right.

One of the revisions to this book is that the dosages of bio-identical progesterone continue to increase. We are now seeing doses of 400 mg to 800 mg per day of natural progesterone being administered routinely with good effects.

One reason for treatment failures in the past was our hesitation to increase the progesterone dose. It was just too low and we were playing it too safe. Now, we routinely increase to 400 mg – 800 mg/day and starting to see complete resolution of symptoms.

We sill recommend starting low and working your way up as many women do get better on lower doses. But it is comforting knowing that we have considerable latitude in dosing on the upper end with complete safety.

My philosophy remains that we should use the lowest possible dose of any hormone supplement that resolves symptoms and not try to be overly aggressive. Time is on our side. Don't be in a big hurry to jump to the higher doses when a lower dose may take care of business completely.

Don't forget that during pregnancy there is up to 100 times more progesterone circulating around in a woman's body than the dosage that we are administering to cure migraines.

Partial Response?

What if you tried taking the recommended dosage of 50 mg twice a day for two or three months and your headaches are less frequent and/or less intense, but still present? Simple – just increase the dose.

The formula is to incrementally add 50 mg of progesterone every couple of months until the headaches are gone - up to a maximum daily dose of 400 – 800 mg/day.

So, if you are one of those women who've been taking progesterone for two or three months and have received a "partial response", here is what you should do:

Beginning the following month, start adding an additional 50 mg of progesterone to your daily dose. So your next increment would be 50 mg in the morning and 100 mg in the evening on days 15 -28 for menstruating women and daily for post-menopausal women (everybody else). Try that for two months and see what happens.

After two more months have passed, if the headaches are improving, but still not gone completely, you may increase the dose again. Add an additional 50 mg of progesterone. So now it would be up to 100 mg two times a day (morning and evening). Again, progesterone should be taken on days 15 – until the first day bleeding for menstruating women and every day if you are post menopausal (category 2).

When we get to this level, I usually put menstruating women on 50 mg, just once a day, on days 1 – 14 as well. To clarify, menstruating women will take 50 mg of progesterone on days 1- 14 and then 100 mg of progesterone, two times daily, during days 15 – until first day of bleeding. Keep in mind that it takes about 6 months of partial responses to get to this level. Most menstruating women never need to worry about this.

One situation we encounter often is that menstruating women who are taking most of their doses in the second half of their cycle are willing to take progesterone every day to get rid of the migraines because that usually works.

Note that taking progesterone in the first half of your menstrual cycle acts as a contraceptive, of sorts, and inhibits ovulation (this is not an endorsement to use this strategy as a birth control pill). In the short run, a menstruating woman can take a level dose of progesterone every single day to rid their migraines.

Later, we can back off the progesterone administration in the first half of the cycle when the woman wants to get pregnant. This strategy works most of the time.

It is mentioned elsewhere, but I will say it again, that it is quite safe to take progesterone during pregnancy. After all, natural levels of progesterone rise a 100 fold beyond anything we are giving you. Because of the massive amounts of progesterone that your own body produces during pregnancy, it doesn't make any sense to take bio-identical supplements beyond 10 weeks or so.

You can email us at: help@migraine-headaches-information.com if you have questions. Keep in mind we get hundreds of emails a day and we will try to get back to you in a couple of business days to answer your questions.

Breast Fullness:

Some women will experience breast fullness or soreness when they start taking progesterone. This is especially true for the higher dosages. Don't worry, this is a normal response and should go away in a few weeks or sooner.

If the breast fullness is just too painful and/or there are other symptoms like ankle swelling (water retention) or worsening of pre-existing PMS symptoms, then it could be because we started the progesterone dose too high.

If this is the case, then it could be because your body is so deficient in progesterone that our starting dose was too high and your body actually converted some of it into estrogen, which worsens the situation.

If this happens, then lower the progesterone to just 50 mg taken only in the evening. Try this for a couple of months. Then you can work up from there depending on the response of your migraines.

The goal is to find the smallest dose that will make your migraine headaches go away.

What If Your Migraines Get Worse Temporarily?

Just like the breast fullness discussion above, some women are so deficient in progesterone that they actually get worsening of the migraines when starting this dosage regimen. If that happens, just back off to one 50 mg progesterone capsule in the evening.

Then you will need to let your body adapt to the new amounts of progesterone circulating around. You will likely have to increase the dosages over time to make your migraines go away completely.

There is one other comment on why your migraines get worse temporarily. Remember the Estrogen Withdrawal Theory I mentioned earlier in this book? Sometimes, as a last ditch measure, I will recommend the administration of bio-identical estrogen during the worst headaches days of your cycle and some women get better.

I am not an advocate of giving estrogen except for menopausal symptoms but as a final measure, we have gotten improvement even if we don't quite understand why.

Other Medications:

Simplicity is always best. If you are taking any other medications, for any other reason, continue to take them as usual. The addition of progesterone should not affect any other prescription or non-prescription medication you are currently taking. (Except for birth control pills. You will need to get off of those as outlined above.)

The reason why I don't recommend changing any of your medications is simply based on the fact that we don't want to change more than one variable at a time. As a general rule, the body does not like change, so we keep it simple by just adding or subtracting one component at a time.

Premarin® vs. PremPro®

If you are currently taking hormone replacement therapy for hot flashes or night sweats in the form of Premarin® or other similar estrogens, you should stay on them. There is no need to discontinue any other hormone (unless it contains the synthetic Provera® component like PremPro®). This is the same artificial progestin found in birth control pills.

If you are taking PremPro®, then this can be changed to just Premarin® without the "Pro". **An even better idea is to substitute a bio-identical estrogen for the Premarin** (which is not human estrogen). But just like the women on birth control pills, you must get off the PremPro®. Otherwise, your migraines will not go away.

Because we are dealing with prescriptions here, you will need your doctor's cooperation on this. However, with all the bad press on PremPro®, I doubt any doctor will have a problem changing PremPro® back to just Premarin®.

Premarin® vs. Bio-Identical Estrogen

In the last year we have become more aggressive in getting women off Premarin® and other synthetic or non-human estrogens and replacing them with bio-identical estrogen.

The manufacturers of our recommended bio-identical progesterone, Progest50, also make a bio-identical estrogen, called Estro325. This is an estrogen cream which we endorse. It can be substituted for Premarin®.

The dosage equivalence of Premarin® with Estro325 is as follows:

One scoop of Estro325 = .325mg of Premarin®
Two scoops of Estro325 = .625mg of Premarin®
Four scoops of Estro325 = 1.25mg of Premarin®

Go to the information site, www.1-Menopause.com for more information about dosing estrogen and menopausal symptoms.

Menopause and Progesterone Administration

Speaking of estrogen, one observation we have made is that some women who are peri-menopausal and on the brink of full-fledged menopausal symptoms of hot flashes, night sweats and vaginal dryness, will begin experiencing their first true menopausal symptoms after beginning progesterone.

The reason is that progesterone is a partial estrogen blocker. Since estrogen deficiency causes menopausal symptoms, we can induce this by adding progesterone.

Note this occurs ONLY in women who are on the brink of menopause.

If this should happen, all we do is add a little bio-identical estrogen and the menopausal symptoms go away. We continue to maintain progesterone to keep the migraines at bay.

IUD's and Implants

If you are on any IUD's with medication in them or an implant like Norplant, those need to be removed. These are essentially identical to birth control pills in their effects. You will not get better until these are removed.

Some IUD's do not have any medication embedded within them. These are the old fashioned copper IUD's. If this is what you have, then they can stay.

Anti-Depressants:

As much as I dislike anti-depressants, if you are already on them (most women with migraines are already taking them, unfortunately), continue to take them as before. Go ahead and start the progesterone as instructed as we change nothing else on your medication regimen.

Over time, as your migraines disappear and never return, *then* you can discontinue the anti-depressants. Again, let your doctor manage the discontinuation process for these drugs, as many of them need to be slowly weaned off of, rather than abruptly stopped. Your doctor should be happy to do this for you as you no longer need these drugs anymore.

Special Situations:

If you follow my program strictly, your migraines should go away after a couple of cycles, or about 60 days. Hence, my reference to getting cured in 60 days on my website. Don't be surprised, however, if you should experience an occasional breakthrough migraine, possibly once or twice a year.

For some reason, we do come across some women whose migraines will breakthrough, despite adhering pretty well to my program. If this happens, do NOT stop the program. Continue taking the progesterone under my recommendations. Do not lose the faith! – and stay with the program.

You will notice, that if you do have a "breakthrough" migraine, that it is milder and shorter than what you experienced before. Not everyone will get another migraine but occasionally some patients do.

Timing Matters!

Sometimes we *can* explain why someone might get a breakthrough migraine. Timing matters! When the recommendation says to begin on day 15, I mean you start taking the progesterone on day 15, not day 16. Starting one day late makes a difference. I have observed mild migraines when women are only one or two days behind schedule.

Keep a close record of your menstrual calendar. Day one is the first day of bleeding. Day 15 is exactly two weeks later. Don't miss it. If you cannot remember, it is better strategy to take your progesterone a day early rather than a day too late. There is no such thing as too much progesterone. There is definitely such a thing as insufficient progesterone, however.

Your Cycle and How it Responds to Stress

Another observation is that your menstrual cycle is vulnerable to outside stimuli that can change the cycle. For example, excessive stress, infections and even things like travel (especially airplane and particularly when crossing several time zones at once). Going to the mountains with an elevation in altitude can alter the menstrual cycle.

Another example is every winter we have an upsurge in migraines. The cold weather does not help. Catching the flu almost always triggers a migraine no matter how good you are with the treatment program.

One interesting observation we have made is the relationship of travel with migraines. For some reason there is a tendency to get a migraine about three or four days after traveling, especially by air. The airport experience apparently has gotten so stressful that it must be significantly affecting the body.

My theory on why a stressful situation results in a migraine a few days later concerns the body's ability to contain stress. Stress is a real physiologic condition where your adrenal glands produce adrenaline during the acute hyper stress phase.

But when the stressful event fades away, i.e. you finished your travel or getting over the flu, your body stops making adrenaline and starts to relax. Boom! That is when you get the migraine.

Why is this? The theory is because your body is probably deficient in cortisol, which is another hormone your adrenal gland makes that circulates around longer and is slower acting in response to stress.

Most women that I have treated have been so stressed out over a couple of decades that their adrenal glands are worn out and just quit making cortisol hormones to a sufficient level that protects the body from longer term stress.

Your Cycle and How it Responds to Progesterone

Cycles can be unpredictable at times when we begin supplementation with natural progesterone. There are three possible outcomes: no change in your cycle (most women), an early (or heavier) period, or a delayed (or no) period.

Fortunately, most women's periods do not change when we add progesterone. Some do, however. We rarely get complaints for the delayed (or no) period. We do get complaints from women whose periods arrived much quicker or heavier than usual.

Why does this happen? For those women whose periods are delayed or don't come at all, it is likely that they are extremely deficient in estrogen. The addition of progesterone simply prevents the final shedding process and hence, a late or very minimal period.

For those women who experience an early or heavy period, it is likely they have excessively high amounts of circulating estrogen. Then we add progesterone, the uterus was previously more developed from high estrogen and becomes bloodier and sheds sooner.

It is difficult to predict who will fall into which category. Admittedly it is trial and error. Fortunately, time is on our side and the body seems to adjust to the new amounts of progesterone that we administer and cycles do seem to smooth out in time, but it may take 4-6 cycles.

Effect of Prescription Medications on Migraines

Prescription medications, especially steroids and even some antibiotics can lengthen, but more likely shorten the cycle. Finally, I have seen injected steroids, like pain shots or epidural steroid injections, which have caused premature menstrual periods.

Anything that changes your menstrual cycle also changes the hormones that affect it. Therefore, a possible breakthrough migraine can occur in each of the above scenarios. The best you can do is just to follow your calendar as best as you can. If there is a change in the cycle, then react accordingly and start the progesterone on the **new** day 15.

A breakthrough migraine may occur anyway, but if you can minimize the external stimuli that keep affecting your cycle, it should iron out in a couple of months. Whatever you do, <u>do not stop the program</u>!

One observation we have made is that the combination of stopping the Pill and beginning progesterone supplementation can cause a short term worsening of your migraines. Fortunately, this will smooth out over a few cycles once the Pill's toxins clear out.

Following the program means that you will be taking bio-identical progesterone for the rest of your life. This is the intention and not a problem. Progesterone is not addictive in any way. You can get off any time. Your body will wash out of the added natural progesterone in just a few days.

But your body will soon revert back to its old ways of being deficient in progesterone. Eventually, your condition will revert back to the old days of frequent migraines and other problems, just like it was before you started taking progesterone supplementation. This is just simple physiology at work.

Pills vs. Creams:

Another delivery system besides taking medications by mouth is the skin (topical application). The problem with skin administration of progesterone (or any other medication) is the extreme variation in absorption through the skin. The skin varies tremendously in its absorption properties in different parts of the body and even in the identical place during the same day.

The reason why the skin is so variable has to do with temperature, whether the skin sub-surface blood vessels are wide open or mostly closed, the amount of sweat and sweat glands. Furthermore, it is very difficult to apply the same amount of cream consistently from a tube.

There is a great deal of variation of product density within the tube with some portions of the tube being very high concentration and other portions being almost completely taken up by fillers.

This is worsened by the fact that creams are difficult to manufacture from one lot to another with any consistency. Few batches of creams are exactly alike. From a manufacturing perspective, it is extremely difficult to get the same cream mixture and consistency each and every time. A batch made last month may be as much as 20% off from one made today.

I have already done the research on cream absorption. Many cream advocates say that the skin is superior in absorption over oral administration because the liver will remove much of the oral dose but the skin does not have to worry about that.

Yes, the skin does absorb chemicals quite well. But the problem is the predictability of how much your skin will absorb versus a known amount by mouth. Your skin never absorbs the same way twice.

Finally, the FDA has some archaic rules preventing cream manufacturers from making a dense enough cream to really help. As a result, to achieve therapeutic doses from a cream, a woman must literally take a bath in the cream.

This is extremely inconvenient, not to mention quite expensive as you end up spending three or four times what was advertised.

The end result is that topical (via skin) dosages vary all over the map and consistency is virtually impossible to maintain. The body will see wild variations in progesterone coming at it and this may actually worsen the condition. In contrast, oral administration is easy, convenient, predictable and safe.

Pills are much easier to take, more convenient to use, and easier to manufacture in a consistent fashion. As a result, blood levels of progesterone are more consistent and predictable.

Oral medications are more predictable in their absorption. Yes, I am fully aware that ALL oral medications are subject to the "first-pass effect" from the liver.

Basically, about 90% of any oral medication, including hormones, are metabolized in the liver and removed from circulation. We know that and have planned the dosage accordingly. That remaining 10% is the desired end result we want.

If a particular oral dose is not effective, then we just increase the dose until it works. Easy. No guess work. No mess.

A Side Note About Estrogen Creams

Having said all of the above about pills and creams, we do recommend a cream when it comes to bio-identical estrogen supplementation. Note that we do not recommend estrogen except for treatment of menopausal symptoms. But when we do recommend an estrogen, it is in a cream form.

Why? Because one study came out earlier this year showing that oral estrogen tended to increase some measurable markers of inflammation versus cream. So for estrogen administration only, we do grudgingly recommend a cream form over oral. For progesterone, we recommend oral use.

THE SOURCES: Finding The Products – Quickly and Easily

A. For Women

For women there are more options than for men. Obtaining the above recommended dosages of progesterone can be done in a variety of ways. They vary in how much you wish to pay and what kind of extra services you desire.

OPTION 1:

Perhaps the best and most thorough means of getting the right treatment and dosages of progesterone is to go to one of the boutique medical clinics that some of my more enterprising colleagues have established. These clinics advertise themselves as wellness, natural medicine, natural hormones, women's health, anti-aging or some similar marketing measures.

You may have seen some advertising for these clinics on billboards or in your local suburban home type of magazines that target high income demographic groups or a magazine in the seat pocket of an airline seat. These boutique practices do not accept insurance but gladly accept your credit card in the amounts near $4000 just to get in the door.

Of course, for your $4000, you get to sip tea from fine china in the reception area, sit on fine furniture on the oriental rugs placed on top of hardwood floors and gaze at some really nice artwork on the walls.

The doctors and staff treat you like royalty and you have a pleasant experience. At the end of the day, you will have the world's most expensive progesterone dosage program, but it works.

Here is the link to perhaps the finest boutique clinic in America that can do this: www.hotzehwc.com

OPTION 2:

You can fly down and come to my clinic and we will do a complete consultation and physical examination. Simply send an email to info@migraine-headaches-information.com or call 281-962-4264 and we will be more than happy to see you in the clinic.

Compared to Option 1 above, my office does not have the fine china, the oriental rugs or the nice artwork. But by the time you finished the initial visit and all of the myriad items that go with it, you would still be paying nearly $2000 from your credit card and insurance is not accepted. Please note that this covers only the doctor visit portion. You still have to obtain your supply of progesterone elsewhere.

Obviously our clinic accountant would love for you to come on down to Houston and visit us. But there are more practical methods than this.

My goal is to spread the word on proper treatment of migraine headaches to as many women worldwide as possible. Keeping this information and treatment reserved exclusive to only the very wealthy is not my idea of accomplishing this.

However, some people just enjoy spending money and we will accept it, but there are better options.

OPTION 3:

Another option is to see if your regular doctor would be willing to write a prescription for the progesterone dosages noted above. Very few doctors on the planet know how to manage bio-identical hormones, particularly when it comes to migraine headaches.

My observation is that most mainstream medical doctors have a) never heard of bio-identical progesterone and would try to write you a prescription for Provera® instead, or b) lecture you on his perception of the "danger" of using natural hormones instead of his comfort zone of prescription drugs created by big drug companies with their myriad of side effects.

Most people do have a good relationship with their doctor. After all, anyone with migraine headaches has likely visited their doctor on numerous occasions and had a number of phone calls as well.

The problem is even if your doctor writes out a prescription for bio-identical progesterone in the recommended dosages, you still have to buy it from a compounding pharmacist. That gets expensive.

Compounding pharmacies, by definition, create just one prescription at a time for a specified patient. They make it by hand with no automation and it is slow, tedious and very expensive. Before my clinic found an alternate means of obtaining bio-identical progesterone, I had no choice but to work with compounding pharmacies in my area.

A typical compounding pharmacy will charge a minimum of one US dollar per capsule, regardless of the dose or even the drug they put in it. The manual labor to make it overwhelms all other costs. So a prescription for 60 capsules in a bottle runs a minimum of US$60.

I remember only a couple of years ago when a capsule was "only" 80 cents a capsule – and we thought that was high. I see more and more compounding pharmacies headed towards the US$1.10 - $1.25 per capsule range now with no end in sight.

The pharmacies must be thinking that they have a monopoly on the creation of natural hormones and believe they can raise the price indefinitely until people start complaining about it more. Little do they know about how the marketplace responds to the need for women to have high quality and low cost natural hormones.

Fortunately, we found a better and far less expensive option that enables you to bypass seeing your doctor and you can obtain natural progesterone for a fraction of the cost that you would pay otherwise.

OPTION 4:

A final option, as well as the simplest and least expensive method, is to find a progesterone product that accomplishes all of my criteria: Oral administration, pure quality, easily shipped, convenient to use, inexpensive and no need for a prescription. We finally found a way around the expensive compounding pharmacy source of natural hormones.

Frankly, we got tired of dealing with the tactics of compounding pharmacies. My patients were facing price increase after price increase, so we started searching around for other options to get them their progesterone.

After a great deal of searching around and research, I have found one progesterone product that satisfies all of the necessary criteria. This is the only non-prescription form of oral progesterone on the planet as far as we can tell.

It can be shipped to you in the exact dose of progesterone (50mg or 100mg) in capsule form. The really good news is that you can get a month's supply of progesterone (for a menstruating woman) for about US$15 and you don't need to see a doctor or get a prescription. You can just order it off the internet.

Once we found this supplier, we started ordering it for our own clinic patients. Since we use so much of it ourselves, I investigated this product and had their progesterone tested in a quality control lab for verification that it was:

a) TRUE bio-identical to human progesterone
b) Actually contains 50 mg (or 100mg) of progesterone within each capsule.

 It passed in both categories.

You can order it off the manufacturer's website at www.progest50.com .

Another feature I like about option #4 is that it comes in 50 mg or 100 mg capsules. I always work in 50 mg increments when it comes to dosage changes and this makes it very convenient.

We have been very pleased with this supplier. American customers receive their orders in a few days and international orders are received in a couple of weeks or so. They tell us they have shipped to 34 countries. The United Kingdom, Canada, Australia and New Zealand are the most frequent countries they ship to, outside of the U.S.

Shipping charges are not very expensive. Canada imposes a customs tax. The U.K. and Australia will occasionally delay a shipment for several weeks. We hear that they will not ship to Germany or the Ukraine.

I get e-mails from my international customers wondering if they can get this progesterone product in their home country. So far, we have not heard of any problems with them receiving their orders in any country except for Germany and the Ukraine.

Some further comments on this particular product, Progest 50:

Here is how the $15/month cost is calculated: You have to purchase the "buy 3 get 2 free" offer from the Progest50 internet site. This costs about US$150 for five bottles. Each bottle contains 60 capsules. Assuming that a menstruating woman takes two capsules daily for half the month, each bottle works out to a two month supply. Five bottles then lasts 10 months, or $15/month.

Non-menstruating women taking a daily Progest50 dose would be twice as much or US$30/month.

The bottle also has a lot of legal language that I have to comment on. Keep in mind that the manufacturer is in America and this label is obviously written by a lawyer, not a doctor. Welcome to the legal climate in America.

The instructions on the bottle tell you to take one capsule two times daily. That's fine, but go back to my instructions on dosages and look up what you need to do if there is a partial response. Be sure and print out my chapter on Dosages and Administration.

The label also says it is not for men or for individuals under 18 years. I agree about the men part, but we do have 13 and 14 year old girls taking it as per my recommendations.

It also talks about not taking it if you are trying to get pregnant, already pregnant or nursing. That is lawyer talk – you can ignore that part. We actually encourage this to women who are trying to get pregnant or are already pregnant.

I also recommend it during nursing because a woman who has just delivered a brand new baby will have a significant chance of post-partum depression, not to mention the return of migraine headaches. So we do use it then.

Finally, the label advises you not to take it if you are using various forms of birth control pills or patches. I agree. You should stop all birth control pills in the manner that has been discussed above.

A Word About Those Progesterone Creams

Many of you are already using a progesterone based cream. I get a lot letters asking if you can continue using them.

As already discussed above, progesterone creams are relatively ineffective. Since so many of you who are using them STILL get migraine headaches – that only underscores their failure to help in this situation.

You might believe simply increasing the amount of cream will alleviate your migraines. Sorry – that won't work. Here's why:

- **Dosages:** First, you have no idea what dosages you're using because it requires an enormous amount of cream to reach a therapeutic level. By that time you're literally taking a bath in the stuff - with all of the hassles that scenario conjures up.

- **Potency:** Don't forget about the manufacturing problems we talked about. Cream manufacturers don't tell you about the variability of hormones within different batches, much less within the same tube. Skin absorption also varies widely. While skin does absorb chemicals quite well, it never absorbs the same way twice. On those days when skin absorption isn't quite up to par, you run the very real risk of a breakthrough migraine headache.

- **Convenience:** Face it – creams are messy, smelly and don't exactly feel great on the skin either. Which would you rather do: Plaster yourself with viscous gunk – or swallow a convenient pill? (That's an easy choice!)

- **Cost:** Finally, creams multiply the cost three or four fold. The preparation you thought was such a bargain can end up costing you US$80 - $100 per month. Not so cheap anymore – is it?

MAGNESIUM SUPPLEMENTATION

Supplementing with magnesium is important because of the synergistic or additive effects we see when combined with your natural progesterone. Extensive discussion of adding magnesium has already been mentioned above in the "*The Secret Mineral that Will Boost the Effectiveness of Your Program and What No Pharmacist Will Tell You about It*" chapter.

Magnesium supplements are manufactured in a myriad of formulations and products. The most common magnesium supplement product you will see at any pharmacy or health food store is in the form of magnesium oxide.

I have already discussed magnesium oxide above and how ineffective it is. You need a superior chemically compatible magnesium compound for your body.

My favorite is a combination of magnesium compounds ending in "ates":

- Magnesium aspartate,
- Magnesium gluconate,

- Magnesium glycinate,
- Magnesium stearate,
- And/or magnesium citrate

As a service to our patients, my staff and I did the field work and research to find the very best magnesium product that met the necessary criteria: multiple "ates", high quality, convenient, and inexpensive. There are hundreds, if not thousands of magnesium products out there and we found the very best one we could recommend for you.

It is called Mag100 and is manufactured by Natural Living, headquartered in Las Vegas, Nevada. Usually, a magnesium product, if it has an "ate" in it will just have one kind. This Mag100 actually has *three*:

- Magnesium aspartate,
- Magnesium gluconate,
- And magnesium glycinate

We actually toured the manufacturing plant. This is where the workers are wearing NASA-like space suits inside the "clean rooms" where the pills are made. It reminded me of the same plant manufacturing quality that the computer chip manufacturers use.

An independent lab has already verified the batch for quality composition.

Mag100 comes in quantity of 60 tablets with each tablet weighing in at 100 mg each. At three times a day dosage, one bottle works out to a one month supply.

The best part is the price – only US$12 per bottle – if you buy their 5-bottle offer, or US$13 per bottle, if you buy their 3-bottle offer. Either way, it is a good deal.

The same people that make Mag100 also make another recommended product - Progest50 (see discussion above). If you buy both products off their website at the same time, the shipping price drops considerably for the second product.

The Natural Living people really have their act together. They make good products (which I have tested in my practice and in the lab) and they packaged some good deals with very reasonable shipping charges.

Over the years, I have come to rely on Natural Living to manufacturer some unique products to my specifications at my request for my patients. You will notice that they now make several of my recommended products.

I used to send my patients to multiple manufacturers and they were bouncing around like in a pinball machine. Natural Living has simplified this process by making the same, quality products for a cheaper price and better service. It is hard to argue with that.

They can ship anywhere in the world – and are especially good at shipping to the U.S., U.K., Canada, Australia and New Zealand.   If you need to look them up on the internet, their website address is www.progest50.com and order directly off their site.

I need to make a couple of comments about international shipping. We get feedback from our readers on all these issues and you need to be aware that some countries have customs duties on imported products. Canada slaps a customs duty on just about every parcel that enters the country.

We have also noticed that the U.K. and especially Australia may hold onto parcels that contain 5 or more bottles (of the same product) for 6 to 8 weeks before releasing them – and then charge a customs tax on top of that.

Recommended Dosage for Magnesium chelates:

Take three tablets per day, divided into morning, lunch and evening, ideally. You can also take (like I do) two tablets in the morning and one in the evening.

Neptune Krill Oil Supplementation

Supplementing with Neptune Krill Oil (NKO) is important because of the synergistic or additive effects we see when combined with your natural progesterone. Extensive discussion of adding NKO has already been mentioned above in the *"Neptune Krill Oil – Natures Remedy from the Sea"* section.

There are a number of Neptune Krill Oil preparations on the market. Our favorite, by far, is a form of NKO that not only naturally packages the omega-3 fatty acids into a phospholipid molecule carrier that makes absorption three times better than standard fish oils, but also contains added astaxanthin, a very powerful anti-oxidant.

Neptune Krill Oil is also 47 times more potent as an anti-oxidant than standard fish oil. As you can see, NKO is clearly superior to fish oil. With the addition of natural astaxanthin, which is six times more potent than fish oil, the final product is very effective.

Where to Get Neptune Krill Oil

After doing extensive searching and watching results, my recommendation for the best product on the market can be found by ordering from Rejuvenation Science online at http://KrillOil.PMScure.com . If you click directly on this link, you will be directed to a VIP area for my patients and become entitled to a 10% discount off their retail price.

Rejuvenation Science is clearly the most effective formulation. There are cheaper generics of Neptune Krill Oil out there, but they are less effective.

Recommended Dosage:

The recommended dosage is to take one gel cap twice daily. NKO by itself is insufficient to cure your migraines. You should take it in combination with the progesterone, magnesium iodine and Vitamin D.

Iodine Supplementation

This is the fourth out of five recommendations. Iodine is critical in thyroid function. Most of the planet is deficient in iodine. Most women with migraines are either frankly hypothyroid or on the brink of being hypothyroid, despite "normal" thyroid blood tests.

As the chapter on iodine earlier in this back points out, iodine supplementation is critically important.

Recommended Dosage:

12.5 mg/day of an iodine/iodide combination plus Vitamin B2, Vitamin B3 and Selenium.

50 mg/day of the above combination for people with thyroid auto-antibodies.

You should take it in combination with the progesterone, magnesium, Krill Oil and Vitamin D.

You can get it at www.IodinePlus.com . This particular product was custom designed for my specifications by the Natural Living people. It has a combination of iodine, iodide, selenium and vitamins B2 and B3. I think it is the world's most perfect thyroid enhancing supplement.

Vitamin D Supplementation

This is the last of my recommendations for first-line treatment of migraine headaches. As the earlier chapter on Vitamin D states, we are all deficient in Vitamin D3.

Vitamin D is not very "sexy" and is passed over by mainstream medicine. The critical importance is now being worked out as something incredibly vital to your long term health.

The recommended doses continue to increase in size. As little as two years ago, only 400 IU's were the standard recommended dose. Now, it is 5000 IU's per day.

Where to Get Vitamin D

Our friends who manufacture Progest50 have also undertaken to make this relatively new product in this dose of 5000 IU's. I cannot find another manufacturer who will make this size. Others, no doubt, will follow in the future.

If you have already been to the Progest50 website you seen their product display for their D5000 brand of Vitamin D. Alternatively you can go to www.VitaminD5000.com . All of these links go to the same page, which is: www.Progest50.com .

Other Supplements

Before I close, let me comment that regardless of your migraine status, that you (and your family – everyone should be taking these) should be taking the following supplements:

- Multivitamins (with large amounts of B vitamins – my favorite is Maximum Vitality). Source: http://doctor.rejuvenation-science.com/andrewjones1/

- Krill Oil - this is the latest and best version of omega-3 oil (Source: http://KrillOil.PMScure.com)

- Vitamin C – at least 3000mg per day

- Calcium – at least 1000 – 1500mg per day

- Magnesium chelates – see prior recommendations: 300 mg/day (source: www.Progest50.com)

- Folic Acid – 400 mcg/day

- Vitamin E – 400 IU's/day

- Vitamin D - 5000 IU's/day
  Source: www.Progest50.com

- Probiotics – Primal Defense – 6 per day
  Source: Whole Foods grocery stores

- Kefir – 8 – 16 ounces/day

We recommend other supplements in other specialty situations, but that is beyond the scope of this book.

Summary of Recommendations:

1. Progesterone – 50 mg, twice daily (or days 15 – first day of bleeding if menstruating) Source: www.Progest50.com

2. Magnesium Chelates – One tablet, three times a day
   Source: www.Progest50.com

3. Krill Oil - this is the latest and best version of omega-3 oil
   Source: http://KrillOil.PMScure.com

4. Iodine – 12.5 mg/day (up to 50 mg/day)
   Source: www.Progest50.com

5. Vitamin D – 5000 IU/day
   Source: www.Progest50.com

B. For Men

Unfortunately, men have very few options to get testosterone. As mentioned before, the Anabolic Steroids Act effectively criminalized possession of testosterone outside of a doctor's prescription for a Schedule III drug. This is the case for Americans, but pretty much most countries around the world now have laws concerning anabolic steroids.

OPTION 1:

So, if a man wants to eliminate his migraine headaches and wants to use the recommended doses of testosterone, he has no choice but to go to the $4000 boutique clinic doctors and pay up. Those clinics will be more than happy to supply him with all of the testosterone he needs.

Unfortunately, it will be virtually impossible to find a regular medical doctor, regardless of how long he has known you, who will prescribe you testosterone. Don't even bother to try. For the doctor, it is like a patient asking him to prescribe cocaine. On most occasions he is not going to do it under any circumstances.

It's sad but true, but testosterone has become so politicized and stigmatized that you will not likely be able to get it without the expensive boutique clinic option (for now).

Don't even think of asking your neurologist to prescribe it. They will laugh you out their office.

The only other option available to men is two-fold, and both come from the same underlying chemistry: precursors.

Precursors are the chemical structures that precede testosterone in their chemical development one or more enzymatic steps before it finally becomes testosterone. The US Congress has outlawed many known precursors to testosterone as part of the Anabolic Steroids Act.

However, one major precursor, DHEA, was specifically exempted from the Act because it is already in the market in huge numbers as a legal dietary supplement. DHEA can then be taken as a dietary supplement in sufficient enough quantities that will be chemically converted into testosterone to help with the migraines.

This is a crude attempt biologically, but it is better than nothing.

OPTION 2:

Therefore, OPTION 2 for men is to take at 200-400 mg a day of DHEA in the form of dietary supplements. DHEA is found in many dietary supplements, vitamin formulations at numerous vitamin and health food stores.

It is usually only manufactured in doses around 25 mg per pill, so doing the math requires taking 8-16 pills per day. This can get very expensive when you do this every day of every month. But since Congress has outlawed the other effective means to cure migraines in men, unfortunately, your legal options are limited.

The Rejuvination Science people have come out with a 100mg size of DHEA. This can be ordered from: http://doctor.rejuvenation-science.com/andrewjones1/

- Did you stop synthetic hormone replacement therapy? (This includes PremPro and all estrogenic drugs).

- Did you remove contraceptive implants or IUD's tainted with synthetic, chemically altered progestins?

Are you taking any other powerful medications that influence hormone levels like:

- Steroids (this includes steroid creams or inhalers)
- Anti-depressant medications
- Blood pressure medications (like beta-blockers, i.e., Inderal)
- Psychotropic drugs (Zyprexa, Seroquel, Risperdol)
- Amphetamines (Ritalin, Adderal)
- Sleep aids
- Valium-like drugs

Have you looked at a great website for information: www.DitchThePill.org ?

If you have done all of the above, then it is officially a treatment failure. It also took several months to get to this point. Now let's discuss this further.

Do You Also Have These Problems?

One observation I have made consistently on the treatment failures is that they tend to have one or more of the following health problems above and beyond migraine headaches. These include:

- Yeast condition
- Irritable bowel syndrome (probably related to yeast)
- Low thyroid
- Chronic Fatigue Syndrome
- Fibromyalgia (probably related to Chronic Fatigue Syndrome)

Stop and Take This On-LineTest

At this point, I want you to stop and take an online test. Go to www.HotzeHWC.com and take their on-line questionnaire. It covers the above topics. Tally up your score and then come back to this chapter when you are finished.

Most of you will score high in one or more of the above categories. Once you have established that, then continue to read on for further explanation and instructions.

Yeast

Yeast is a huge topic all by itself. The terms "yeast" and "Candida" are interchangeable.   Candida are simply multiple strains of yeast. There are probably hundreds of Candida strains that comprise yeast. They are all toxic.

Mainstream medicine virtually totally ignores yeast, but it is epidemic and endemic. Almost every woman on the planet has had a "yeast infection" at one time in her life, so women know what yeast is, even if her doctor doesn't.

Yeast is much more than just a vaginal yeast infection. Yeast is actually a type of mold or fungus. Yeast lives just about everywhere except in extreme dry climates. Even so, yeast still lives INSIDE YOU.

Our bodies are colonized with yeast just like our intestines are colonized with bacteria – some friendly, some harmful. If bacteria can live inside our intestines, why can't yeast? They also live in your sinuses, your vagina and sometimes in your skin, toenails, inner ear and any other place in or on your body.

As babies we are exposed and colonized with yeast (remember diaper rash? – that is yeast). Oral thrush in babies is also yeast. How about those ear infections? Mainstream medicine hands out reams of antibiotics and guess what? We get yeast to colonize the ear canals afterwards.

Yeast are everywhere and we can't do anything about it. But when we take antibiotics or steroids, the balance of power between yeast and bacteria changes. Antibiotics indiscriminately kill off beneficial bacteria which results in an overgrowth of yeast.

Dysbiosis and Irritable Bowel Syndrome

Yeast produce toxins that circulate and cause dozens of strange symptoms. Yeast are responsible for "dysbiosis", which is an overgrowth of yeast in the intestines resulting in gas, bloating, abdominal pain, diarrhea that mainstream medicine calls Irritable Bowel Syndrome (IBS).

Unfortunately, mainstream medicine completely misses the boat on how to effectively treat IBS. They have identified the symptoms but haven't figured out what causes it and definitely have no idea how to cure it. They just throw toxic medications at it.

Yeast are also responsible for chronic sinus conditions, ear infections and many allergies. They are almost always present in people who have resistant migraines.

If you wish to learn more on the subject, a couple of good books to read are: *The Yeast Syndrome* and *The Yeast Connection*. They are available from Amazon's website at the following links:

http://AmazonYeastSyndrome.pmscure.com and http://AmazonYeastConnection.pmscure.com.

Doctors have no idea how to treat IBS or any other yeast condition acquired outside of a hospital. You will need a yeast-killing antibiotic like Diflucan, Nizoral or Sporonox. Nizoral is the least expensive one and works just as well as the others.

You will need to take one of those yeast killers for a LONG TIME - like 6 months. I personally took Sporonox for 8 months in a row. (I had the same thing you did). Doctors will fall out of their chair when you request a 6 month supply of one of these medications, but I speak from experience.

You will also need to take an anti-yeast drug, called Nystatin, three or four times a day that kills intestinal yeast on contact. Nystatin is not absorbed into the bloodstream and stays strictly inside the intestines.

Another major weapon to use against yeast is a class of dietary supplements called "probiotics". Basically these are the "good" bacteria that you need to colonize your intestines. These are the bacteria that help your digestion process.

They are essential to healthy digestion. Good bacteria, like *lactobacillus* species have a symbiotic relationship with us. In exchange for free room and board inside our intestines, they help us digest our foods. It is a win-win relationship.

Unfortunately that relationship gets altered when we introduce antibiotics or steroids into our bodies. Good bacteria help suppress yeast and bad bacteria that want to set up shop inside you. When antibiotics indiscriminately kill off good bacteria and the bad at the same time, not only does that encourage yeast growth, but it also encourages an overgrowth of bad bacteria.

Primal Defense

In order to keep the body's digestive tract well colonized with good bacteria, we recommend probiotics daily. My favorite probiotic is called Primal Defense. It is manufactured by the Garden of Life people and you can get it from health food stores and Whole Foods Markets.

Work up to 6 Primal Defense tablets/day divided into 2 daily doses on an empty stomach. In other words, take three in the morning when you get up and three at night. Do not start taking 6 tablets when you first start. You slowly work up to that level starting with just one a day for a couple of days. Then go to two, then three, etc., until you reach the total of six.

Kefir

Another great product as an add-on to Primal Defense (not in place of it), is a dairy product called Kefir. It is like yogurt, but several times better. Many gastroenterologists consider it to be the world's most perfect food item. I agree. You just cannot get enough of it.

The plain, unflavored version tastes very similar to buttermilk. Many people like it (myself included). If you are not a fan of the unflavored version, try the flavored versions – strawberry, blueberry, vanilla and the like.

Kefir is so mainstream nowadays that many regular grocery stores are starting to carry it. If yours does not, try a health food store.

But don't limit it just for yourself. Your entire family will benefit from the world's most healthy beverage. This also includes your children. (There is even a special line of "kid kefir". The only difference from the adult brand is that it is entirely organic.

Worthless Candida Remedies

Some people describe long holistic yeast (Candida) treatment experiences that involve incredible complex programs from strict diets to "purges". They have usually been on multiple herbal remedies. The diets are impossible to maintain. And nothing has worked.

I have no trouble with diet alterations (reducing the carb intake), or purges, or any of these items. But until you add the yeast killing drugs mentioned above, you will NEVER get rid of the yeast-related problems.

The end result is that until the yeast condition is addressed, your migraine headaches won't budge. So get on your yeast program and once that improves, get back on the migraine treatment program described earlier in this book.

Low Thyroid

If you want to select a "favorite" hormone for both men and women, the hands down choice is thyroid. Why? Because thyroid has a significant role in just about every metabolic or chemical reaction in the body.

Thyroid deals with a huge range of body physiology. It is involved in everything from fat burning to hair growth. Thyroid influences skin moisture and helps develop a child's brain IQ. So thyroid is vitally important, and without it, you will literally shrivel up and die.

The following are some of the major symptoms and signs associated with an under active thyroid:

- Depression
- Weight gain
- Difficulty losing weight
- Low energy - fatigue
- Cold natured
- Ice-cold hands or feet
- Dry skin
- Hair loss (alopecia)
- Slowed thinking, poor concentration
- Brain fog

- Memory problems
- Insomnia, poor sleep
- Waking up exhausted
- Tingling in hands and feet
- Muscle pain
- Edema (swelling in ankles)
- Constipation
- Slow heart rate
- Low blood pressure
- Elevated cholesterol
- Thickened tongue
- Anemia
- Thinned eyebrows
- Slow reflexes
- Cool body temperature

However, frank hypothyroidism is not that common. Most of the time when doctors check blood thyroid levels, they usually come back quite "normal". At this point, the doctor will usually tell you that there is "nothing wrong with you" and writes you a prescription for an anti-depressant medication.

Unfortunately, there are significant testing problems with the typical encounter in the doctor's office when it comes to thyroid:

First, the lab values of "normals" are too wide. In other words, the lab has too many people within the normal range. In my observation, about a third of the population should be in the "abnormal" range, particularly over the age of 30. The laboratories used too large a data base to calculate the normal values for a population.

Another problem is the presence of what is called "auto-antibodies" to your own thyroid hormone. The medical name for this is "Hashimoto's Disease". About a third of all women have thyroid anti-bodies and about a sixth of men have them, too.

This means that your body's immune system has somehow been programmed to attack and destroy circulating thyroid hormone in your own body. So the lab can measure all the thyroid hormone it wants, but the end effect of thyroid is not making it inside the cells of the body to start working.

Finally, and this is crucial – your body's ability to manufacture any hormone peaks around the age of 25. After that, hormone manufacturing capability declines at a rate of about 1% - 3% on an annual basis thereafter.

Mathematically, by the time you reach 40, your hormone production could be down as much as 45%. By your 70th birthday, your hormone production could be just a fraction of what it used to be when you were younger.

This math not only applies to thyroid hormone, but all hormones, including estrogen, progesterone and testosterone, regardless of sex.

The end result is just because your thyroid blood tests were "normal" – don't believe it. There is a very long list of symptoms when your thyroid is under active or deficient.

Add Iodine

In the last year, we have totally changed our recommendations for thyroid treatment. There is a chapter in this book discussing this.

Our first line treatment for thyroid beginning in 2008 is to administer significant supplementation with iodine. I will not repeat everything previously mentioned but you should be taking iodine by the time you get to this chapter on failed treatment.

Add Thyroid Hormone

I frequently add some thyroid hormone to everyone who has intractable migraines, regardless of whether their thyroid blood tests are normal or not.

Where to Get Thyroid?

There are two ways to get thyroid: getting your doctor to write you a prescription for thyroid hormone or get it as a dietary supplement in the form of a thyroid extract.

Convincing your doctor to write a prescription for you is difficult. The problem with this is that most doctors will refuse to do this when you test "normal" on your thyroid blood tests.

There is likely not a single mainstream doctor on this planet who will write a thyroid prescription in the face of "normal" blood tests. Progressive doctors who are familiar with bio-identical hormones write thyroid prescriptions nearly 100% of the time, but generally these doctors are very expensive and do not take insurance.

Just for completeness, if your doctor was agreeable to write the thyroid prescription the next problem is that they will universally give you the wrong kind. Doctors love to prescribe a type of thyroid called "T4" or levothyroxine. The brand names for this include: Synthroid, Levothroid, Levoxyl, and Unithroid.

Although you can get away with these brands about half of the time, I do not recommend any of them. Instead, you need a type of thyroid called "T3" or triiodothyronine. The reason why T3 is preferred over T4 is because T3 is the active form of thyroid in the body's cells.

Many people have difficulty converting their T4 into the T3 form. Therefore, any prescription that is exclusively T4 may not be helpful.

We prefer the prescription Armour thyroid. Armour thyroid is an extract that has a combination of T3 with T4. It is far more effective than the T4-only brands.

It must be Brand Name Only for Armour thyroid. No generics!

The prescription that the doctor should write is:
Armour thyroid –
½ grain by mouth on a daily basis for two weeks. After 2 weeks, increase the dose to 1 grain daily thereafter.

How to Get Thyroid Without a Prescription

If your doctor is unwilling to prescribe you thyroid medication, then you will have to get it yourself. Here's how:

You can get a dietary supplement version of thyroid extract. Order it off the internet. This is very difficult to find, but my favorite thyroid extract that you can get without a prescription can be found at: http://Thyroid.DepressionGoneForever.com

It is called **"Raw Thyroid"**. It is a thyroid extract just like Armour thyroid but in smaller doses so it doesn't fall into a prescription drug category.

It is very inexpensive and easy to use.

Recommended Dosage for Raw Thyroid:

The recommended dosage for Raw Thyroid is to take **one pill twice daily** for the first two weeks. The amount of thyroid extract works out at this dose to the equivalent of a half grain of Armour thyroid.

After two weeks, you can double this dose to **two capsules, twice daily** to become equivalent to the one grain dose of Armour thyroid.

Chronic Fatigue Syndrome/Fibromyalgia

This is another condition that I see that is very common in women who have resistant migraines. I have included both of these conditions together as I believe they are both variations of the same thing.

Chronic Fatigue Syndrome (CFS) is characterized by extreme, profound weakness and fatigue at all times of the day. Some people are so affected that they are almost bedridden. Most people fall into some milder version whereby they run out of gas in the early afternoon. Many people with CFS also have an associated chronic pain condition identical to Fibromyalgia.

Fibromyalgia Syndrome (FMS) is characterized by a chronic pain condition that has numerous tender or trigger points. Mainstream medicine has very specific criteria for diagnosis that requires so many trigger points to qualify. My easy to remember version of FMS is that you have very tender and painful muscles. If someone touches you and you go "ouch", then you have FMS.

People with FMS almost always have a fatigue component strikingly similar to CFS. This is why I maintain that CFS and FMS are basically the variations of the same theme.

Unfortunately, the treatment recommendations for CFS/FMS are very complicated and tedious. I will say the basis in treatment lies in the replenishment of adrenal hormones as well as thyroid. This requires a very detailed step-by-step algorithm that we have developed that goes way beyond the scope of this book.

At this point, my recommendation would be to concentrate on the yeast and thyroid issues before plunging into the CFS/FMS arena. That will be several months of experimentation.

Other Supplements

Before I close, let me comment that regardless of your migraine status, that you (and your family – everyone should be taking these) should be taking the following supplements:

- Multivitamins (with large amounts of B vitamins – my favorite is Maximum Vitality). Source: http://doctor.rejuvenation-science.com/andrewjones1/

- Krill Oil - this is the latest and best version of omega-3 oil (source: http://KrillOil.PMScure.com)

- Vitamin C – at least 3000mg per day

- Calcium – at least 1000 – 1500mg per day

- Magnesium chelates – see prior recommendations: 300 mg/day Source: www.Progest50.com

- Folic Acid – 400 mcg/day

- Vitamin E – 400 IU's/day

- Vitamin D - 5000 IU's/day Source: www.Progest50.com

- Probiotics – Primal Defense – 6 tablets per day Source: Whole Foods grocery store

- Kefir – 8 – 16 ounces/day

We recommend other supplements in other specialty situations, but that is beyond the scope of this book.

Conclusion

I hope this helps for the 20% of women who have tried the bio-identical progesterone treatment and failed to get better. It is extremely likely that you saw many of your other health conditions in this chapter and can now act accordingly.

Conclusion

Well, there you have it. Migraine headaches are more common than anticipated and have overlapping qualities with cluster headaches in men. Migraines are probably intimately related to the menstrual cycle and sex hormones in women. They are a function of a deficiency of sex hormones (testosterone) in men.

The good news for migraine sufferers out there is that based on our historical treatment rates we can cure about 80% of you. Follow my advice above and **you WILL be cured** with no more severe headaches for the rest of your life.

For menstruating women, expect about two menstrual cycles to go by to get the full effect and you should not have any more migraine headaches. So, after about 60 days you should be cured.

For non-menstruating women and for men, your cure results can come somewhat quicker.

As I said before, we have an 80% cure rate. For the remaining 20%, many of them may have headaches caused by something different than sex hormone deficiency, and there is also a small percentage of people with migraines who just don't respond as well to our usual hormone treatment.

Even if you are in the 20% of people whose headaches do not improve, I guarantee that if you follow my program that you will feel better anyway in other areas, both men and women. Also, your headaches will not be as severe as they were before, even if the source is different from what we thought.

The reason is that correcting hormonal imbalances (or deficiencies) will have an overall positive effect on your health and well-being. You will feel better. Your body will function better. You will stay younger longer. It's all good.

So, good luck. Go order your hormones – progesterone for women, testosterone (or DHEA) for men. Don't forget your magnesium, Krill Oil, iodine and Vitamin D. And start feeling better in 60 days.

Andrew P. Jones, M.D.

P.S.

Other books by Dr. Jones:

The Natural Cure to Your Migraine Headaches, 4th Edition
– order from www.Migraine-Headaches-Information.com

The All-Natural Cure to Your PMS
– order from www.PMScure.com

The All-Natural Cure to Your Depression
– order from www.DepressionGoneForever.com

In my practice of treating women, not only have I come across maladies like migraines, but also numerous other problems endemic within the female population.

I have published two other books recently – one on depression and the other on PMS. Both are written in a similar style to this book explaining in common language what these conditions are and how to cure them forever.

To order these books, simply click on the book title link or email my office at: help@WomensHealthInstituteofTexas.com or call 281-962-4264.

Other resource websites:
Birth Control Pill information: www.DitchThePill.org
Menopause information: www.1-Menopause.com
Online hormone questionnaire:
http://www.hotzehwc.com/test/

Disclaimer:

This book represents the views of Dr. Jones alone. It is not intended to allow non-physicians to practice medicine but rather to improve a patient's understanding of their medical condition. Dr. Jones believes that an informed patient can assist better in their own medical care which results in a better outcome for the patient.

This book is not intended for diagnosis but rather to offer information to make you a better informed patient. Discuss any medication changes with your physician prior to making any changes. Please consult your physician for your own personal medical advice.